Vascular Disorders of the Ocular Fundus

A Colour Manual of
Diagnosis

Other 'Colour Manuals in Ophthalmology'

Retinal Detachment

The Eye in Systemic Disease

Uveitis

all by Jack J. Kanski

Contact Lenses in
Ophthalmology

by Michael Wilson and
Elisabeth Millis

Glaucoma

by Jack J. Kanski and
James A. McAllister

Vascular Disorders of the Ocular Fundus

A Colour Manual of Diagnosis

Rodney H. B. Grey,
MA, MB BChir, FRCS, DO, FCOphth

Consultant Ophthalmologist,
Bristol Eye Hospital, Bristol

Butterworths
London   Boston   Singapore
Sydney   Toronto   Wellington

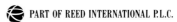 PART OF REED INTERNATIONAL P.L.C.

First published 1991

© Butterworth–Heinemann Ltd, 1991

British Library Cataloguing in Publication Data
Grey, Rodney H. B.
    Vascular disorders of the ocular fundus.
    1. Man. Eyes. Disorders
    I. Title   II. Series
    617.7

ISBN 7506-1033-6

Library of Congress Cataloging-in-Publication Data
Grey, Rodney H. B.
    Vascular disorders of the ocular fundus/Rodney
    H.B. Grey.
        p.   cm. – (Colour manuals in ophthalmology)
    Includes bibliographical references.
    Includes index.
    ISBN 7506-1033-6
    1. Fundus oculi–Blood vessels–Diseases.   I. Title.
    II. Series.   [DNLM: 1. Fundus Oculi.   2. Retinal
    Diseases–diagnosis.
    3. Retinal Diseases–therapy.   4. Retinal Vessels–
    physiopathology.
    WW 270 G844v]
    RE545.G74   1990
    617.7'3–dc20
    DNLM/DLC   90-2226
    for Library of Congress   CIP

Composition by Genesis Typesetting, Laser Quay, Rochester, Kent
Printed in Scotland by Cambus Litho, Glasgow
Bound by Hartnolls Ltd, Bodmin, Cornwall

Preface

The management of vascular diseases of the fundus occupies a large proportion of the work of every general ophthalmologist and particularly those with a special interest in posterior segment problems. This book is designed to be a practical guide to the assessment and treatment of patients with vascular disorders. It is intended to bridge the gap between the basic general textbooks and the comprehensive, multiple volume works. I hope that those studying for higher examinations will find it useful.

A further reading section has been included with each chapter so that readers who wish to explore more deeply can do so. The list of references is not comprehensive but should allow those interested to trace further aspects of retinal disease without difficulty.

My thanks are extended to Terry Tarrant for his drawings, to Mr Ronald Marsh, Mr Edward Schulenburg and Professor John Marshall for the loan of illustrations, to Mrs Gill Bennerson who took most of the photographs and to Mr Jack Kanski for editorial help. I am indebted to the Board of Governors of Moorfields Eye Hospital for kind permission to reproduce figures 6.9, 6.14, 6.20, 6.30, 7.6, 7.8, 8.3 and 10.7. Special thanks go to Mrs Linda Clayton who worked extremely hard on the manuscript.

R.H.B.G.

To Hermione

Contents

1

Normal vasculature of the fundus

Circulation of the globe

The blood supply to the eye is derived from branches of the ophthalmic artery (Figure 1.1). The central retinal artery leaves the ophthalmic artery where it lies inferior to the optic nerve, penetrates the dura infero-medially 12–15 mm behind the globe and runs forwards within the optic nerve to emerge at the lamina cribrosa of the optic nerve head. Here it divides into superior and inferior branches lying on the nasal side of the optic disc and becomes visible ophthalmoscopically. The superior and inferior branches redivide into nasal and temporal arterioles close to the rim of the optic disc and these in turn arborize into second- and third-order arterioles producing the typical vascular pattern of the retina (Figure 1.2). The major retinal vessels lie in the nerve fibre layer of the neuroretina.

The ciliary arteries are composed of multiple short ciliary arteries (up to 20) and a medial and a lateral long ciliary artery (Figure 1.1). They leave the ophthalmic artery just before it divides into its terminal branches, run forward surrounding the optic nerve and penetrate the posterior sclera. Having transversed the sclera the short ciliary arteries immediately divide into multiple small arterioles supplying the choroid and the laminar and prelaminar portions of the optic nerve head via the circle of Zinn. The long ciliary arteries penetrate the sclera on the medial and lateral sides of the optic nerve, continue forwards in the

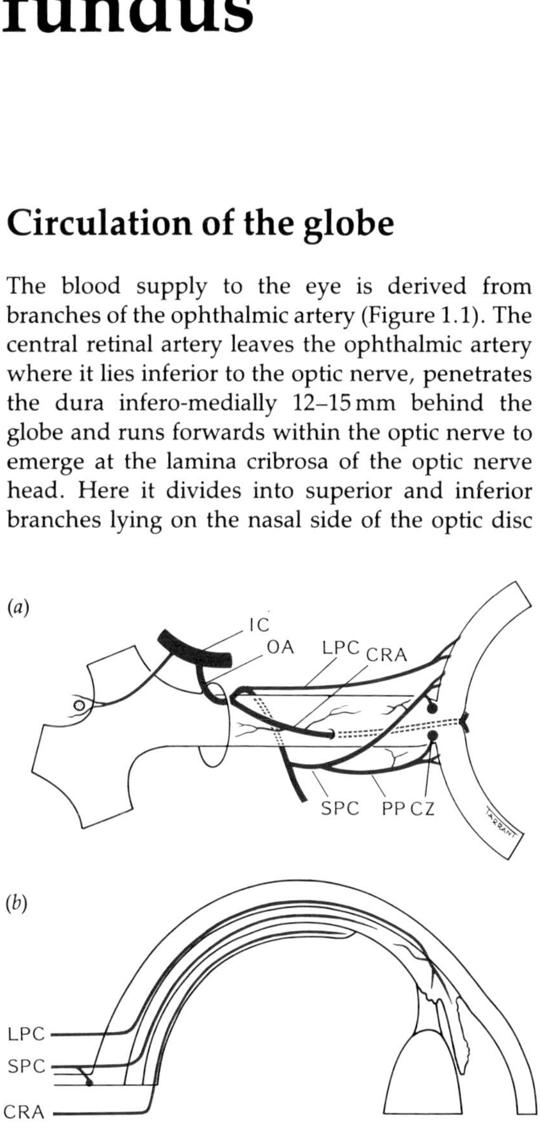

(a)

(b)

Figure 1.1 (*a*) Diagram of arterial supply to the eye in the orbit (from below). IC = internal carotid; OA = ophthalmic artery; SPC = short posterior ciliary artery; CZ = circle of Zinn; CRA = central retinal artery; LPC = long posterior ciliary artery; PP = pial plexus. (*b*) Diagram of arterioles of globe

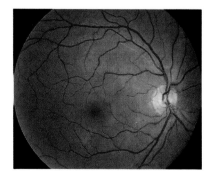

Figure 1.2 Vascular pattern of the normal fundus

1

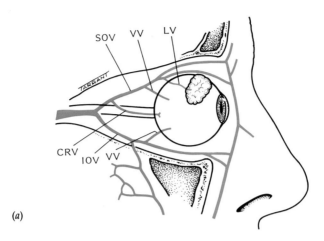

(a)

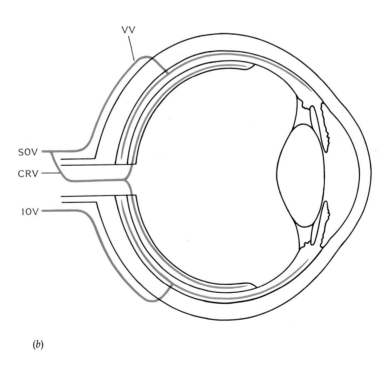

(b)

Figure 1.3 Diagram of venules of globe. SOV = superior ophthalmic vein; IOV = inferior ophthalmic vein; LV = lacrimal vein; VV = vortex vein; CRV = central retinal vein

superficial choroid to the ciliary body where they anastomose with branches of the anterior ciliary arteries. They supply the ciliary body and iris and contribute to the anterior choroidal circulation.

The venous drainage of the retina is via the central retinal vein and its tributaries, which broadly correspond to the arterioles of the retina and optic nerve. The vein emerges from the optic nerve close to the artery, crosses the subarachnoid space and drains into either the superior ophthalmic vein or the cavernous sinus. The choroidal veins do not follow the arterial pattern but collect into four major vortex veins emerging from the sclera between the equator and posterior pole of the globe and drain into the ophthalmic veins (Figure 1.3).

Inner retinal circulation

The branches of the central retinal artery are end arterioles supplying circumscribed territories with no anastomoses to neighbouring arterioles. The vessel walls are composed of a layer of endothelial cells with their basement membrane and a thin muscle coat; there is no internal elastic lamina. The vessel walls are not seen ophthalmoscopically but in some diseases they become visible; in the healthy state only the column of blood can be observed. In spite of some sympathetic innervation there is no known neurological control of retinal arteriolar calibre but the diameter of the vessels can vary according to local metabolic changes or intraluminal pressure alterations.

The retinal capillary bed is composed of an inner and an outer layer, the former at the level of the ganglion cells and the latter in the inner nuclear layer of the retina. Both capillary layers are composed of endothelial cells, basement membrane and mural cells (pericytes). In common with the cerebral capillaries but unlike those of other tissues each endothelial cell forms 'tight' junctions with adjacent cells, producing an impervious barrier to fluid transfer across the capillary wall. This is known as the inner blood–retinal barrier. There is no extracellular space in the neuroretina and, therefore, no extravascular fluid compartment. Around the retinal arterioles there is a narrow zone which is free of capillaries.

Several areas of the retina have variations on the normal capillary bed described above. A zone of approximately 400 μm diameter centred on the foveola has no capillaries – the so-called capillary free zone or foveal avascular zone. In the retinal periphery the layers of the capillaries tend to be less defined and fewer in number. At the optic disc head there is an additional layer of capillaries known as the prepapillary plexus, lying near the surface of the retina and extending into the surrounding nerve fibre layer for 1–2 disc diameters.

The capillary bed of the retina supplies nutrients to and removes metabolites from the innermost layers of the retina, i.e. nerve fibre, ganglion cell, inner plexiform and inner nuclear layers. The photoreceptors (outer nuclear layer) are supplied by the choriocapillaris; the outer plexiform layer lies at the watershed between retinal and choroidal supply (Figure 1.4).

The retinal venules largely follow the pattern of the arterioles, collecting into superior and inferior nasal and temporal branches. The nasal and temporal tributaries join together close to or on the optic nerve forming superior and inferior branches, which in turn join to form the central retinal vein egressing through the lamina cribrosa on the temporal side of the central retinal artery. The retinal veins appear broader than their arteriolar counterparts (diameter ratio 3:2) and their walls are thinner consisting only of an endothelial cell layer and connective tissue. Where a vein crosses an arteriole the vessels share a common adventitial sheath.

Outer retinal and choroidal circulation

The arterial supply to the choroid is derived mainly from the short posterior ciliary arteries except anteriorly where there is a contribution from the long ciliary arteries via the ciliary body. The short ciliary arteries rapidly divide into multiple branches within the choroid forming an extensive broad capillary plexus, the choriocapillaris (Figure 1.4). Unlike retinal capillaries, choroidal capillaries do not have 'tight' junctions and, therefore, are freely permeable to fluid transfer. The choriocapillaris is impermeable to large plasma molecules, such as proteins, and cellular constituents of blood.

The retinal pigment epithelium consists of a monolayer of hexagonal cells. Each cell forms a tight junction (zona occludens) with its neighbours preventing the extracellular fluid of the

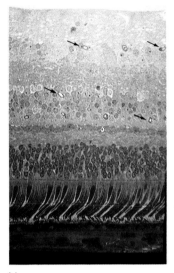

(a)

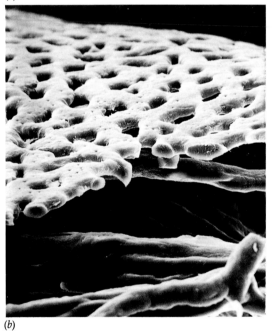

(b)

Figure 1.4 (*a*) Transection of the retina and choroid. The capillaries lie in the nerve fibre and inner nuclear layers (arrows). (*b*) Scanning electron micrograph of the choriocapillaris and underlying larger choroidal vessels (monkey). (Courtesy of Professor John Marshall)

choroid entering the retina, thus forming the outer blood–retinal barrier. The pigment epithelium has an active metabolic pump which transfers fluid across the cell body; the direction of water flow is from the vitreous and neuroretina into the choroid.

The choriocapillaris is a highly vascular structure and provides nutrients to and removes metabolic products from the outer retinal layers, namely the photoreceptors (outer nuclear layer plus rod and cone layer) and the retinal pigment epithelium. These structures have extremely high metabolic rates but, despite this, choroidal blood is less than 20% deoxygenated when it reaches the choroidal veins. It has been postulated that an additional function of the choriocapillaris is to act as a heat regulator maintaining an even temperature for the photochemical and visual processes of the photoreceptors and pigment epithelium.

At the optic disc head there is a variation from the normal choroidal capillaries. The laminar and prelaminar portions of the optic nerve are supplied by the circle of Zinn which surrounds the lamina cribrosa and is derived from choroidal arterioles. The capillaries in this area are, therefore, choroidal in origin but resemble retinal capillaries in that they have tight junctions maintaining the blood–retinal barrier.

Venous blood is collected by the numerous choroidal veins which lead to ampullae and the vortex veins which exit from the sclera. There are usually four vortex veins lying a little posterior to the equator of the globe close to the medial and lateral borders of the superior and inferior recti. However, the position and number of the vortex veins is variable.

Anomalies of circulation

Retinal

In common with other organs of the body, variations in the normal vascular arrangements are not infrequent. Such variations occur as a result of anomalies during embryonal development and do not usually lead to pathological changes. It has been estimated that 10–20% of the population have cilioretinal arteries at the optic disc, i.e. choroidal arteries supplying the retinal circulation

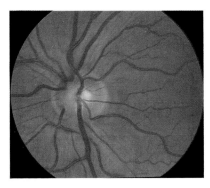

Figure 1.5 Inferonasal cilioretinal artery and nasal venous opticociliary vein

(Figure 1.5). Retinal capillaries supplied from the choroid develop tight junctions.

Other common anomalies include superior branches of arteries or veins serving inferior areas of the retina (or vice versa), congenital arterial or venous tortuosity (Figure 1.6) and also persistence of a hyaloid arterial remnant (Bergmeister's papilla) (Figure 1.6).

More rarely arterial or venous loops at the optic disc may be observed and occasionally arteriolar or venular anastomoses may occur (Figure 1.7). These conditions remain symptomless and are usually discovered by chance.

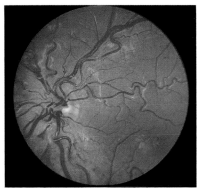

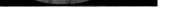

(a)

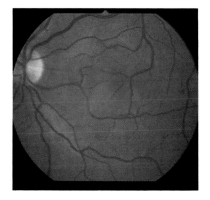

(a)

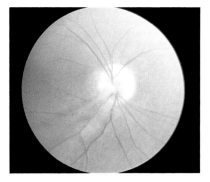

(b)

Figure 1.6 (*a*) Congenital arterial tortuosity. (*b*) Persistent hyaloid artery

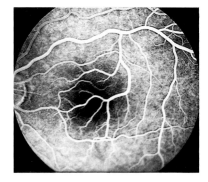

(b)

Figure 1.7 (*a*) Arterio-venous anastomosis. (*b*) Angiogram of (*a*)

Choroidal

In the normal eye the retinal pigment epithelium prevents visualization of the choroidal vessels by ophthalmoscopy. Some individuals, for instance Caucasian children, or the elderly have reduced pigment, and choroidal vessels can be observed particularly in the periphery of the fundus. In patients with albinism (Figure 1.8) the larger choroidal vessels are readily visible over the entire fundus, whereas conditions producing localized atrophy of the pigment reveal the choroid through 'windows' (Figure 1.9).

Congenital absence of the choroidal vessels occurs with a choroidal coloboma (Figure 1.10). Failure of fusion of the developing retinal pigment epithelium produces a lack of the determining factors responsible for choroidal development from the surrounding mesoderm.

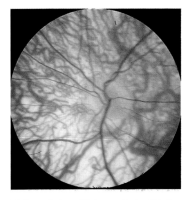

Figure 1.8 Normal choroidal vessels in albinism

Further reading

DUKE-ELDER, S. (1961) *System of Ophthalmology*, Vol. II, Harry Kimpton, London

JAKOBIEC, F. A. (1982) *Ocular Anatomy, Embryology and Teratology*, Harper and Row, New York

RYAN, S. J. (1989) *Retina*, Vol. I, Chapters 7 and 8, C. V. Mosby, New York

WISE, G. N., DOLLEY, C. T. and HENKIND, P. (1971) *The Retinal Circulation*, Harper and Row, New York

WOLFF, E. (1976) *Anatomy of the Eye and Orbit*, H. K. Lewis, London

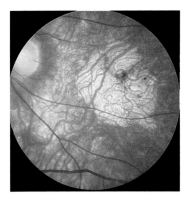

Figure 1.9 Choroidal vessels visible through dystrophic pigment epithelium

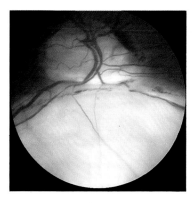

Figure 1.10 Absent choroidal vessels in choroidal coloboma

2

Fundus fluorescein angiography

The technique of fundus fluorescein angiography was first introduced in 1961 and has contributed greatly to the understanding of the retinal circulation and its disorders.

Principles

Substances that fluoresce have the property of absorbing light of one wavelength and emitting light of a different wavelength. Sodium fluorescein, when stimulated by blue light, becomes activated and emits green light (Figure 2.1).

During fluorescein angiography, the xenon flash of a fundus camera produces white light which is passed through a blue exciting filter and thence into the eye. It is reflected from the fundus as a mixture of blue light and green light where fluorescein is present. The emergent mixture passes through a second, barrier filter, which transmits only green and yellow light, and then to a camera plate (Figure 2.2).

Provided the optical properties of the camera and the eye are good and the filters are sufficiently selective to prevent overlap of the exciting and emitting wavelengths, a detailed photograph of the retinal circulation can be obtained. Serial photographs allow a dynamic study of the blood flow through the retina.

Technique

Five millilitres of 20% sodium fluorescein are injected into an antecubital vein; rapid injection results in better quality angiographic pictures than slow injection because a larger bolus of dye enters the retinal circulation.

Serial photographs are taken on black and white film, the type of film depending on the camera characteristics. As the fluorescein enters the eye, exposures are taken approximately every second for 15 s, then with decreasing frequency for 2–3 minutes. Sometimes late exposures at 15 minutes can be useful.

Considerable help in interpreting the processed film can be obtained by stereoscopic photographs. As the pupil requires dilatation for angiography it is often possible to obtain left and right stereoscopic pairs of photographs either by using an image separator or more simply by moving the

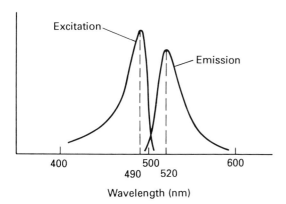

Figure 2.1 Principles of fluorescence

camera slightly to the left and then to the right of the pupil. Assessment of some diseases, particularly ageing macular changes, can frequently be made much easier by stereoscopic pairs of photographs.

To date video angiography has not been greatly successful but image enhancement from intensifiers now available may make this a useful alternative for the future.

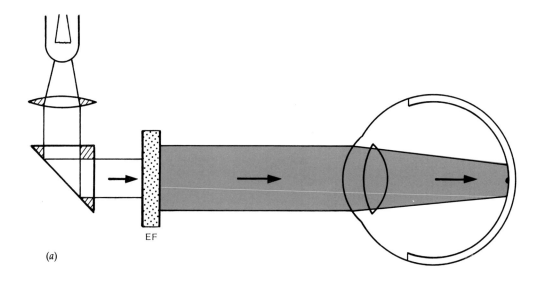

(a)

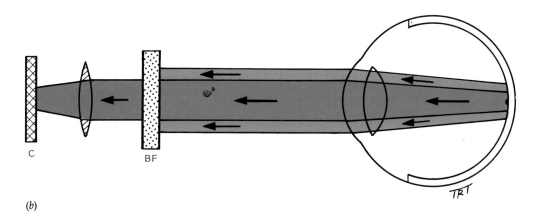

(b)

Figure 2.2 Principles of angiography. (*a*) Excitation filter (EF) passes only blue light into the eye. (*b*) Barrier filter (BF) passes only green light to return to the camera (C)

Alternative techniques

It is not always necessary to record fluorescein angiography on film. Fluoroscopy can be carried out using a similar injection technique as for angiography but observation is by indirect ophthalmoscopy with a blue filter in front of the light source. This can be useful for identifying foci of retinal neovascularization or for examining the far retinal periphery where photography is difficult.

Indocyanine green has been used instead of sodium fluorescein but has not been shown to be superior for retinal vascular changes. This technique has some advantages for choroidal vessel assessment but has proved technically difficult to develop.

The normal angiogram

Fluorescein in the bloodstream is 60% bound to albumin. In the retinal circulation both the bound and unbound fractions remain within the lumen of the blood vessels on account of the inner blood retinal barrier, but in the choroidal circulation the unbound fraction passes through the fenestrations of the choriocapillaris into the extracellular space (Figure 2.3).

In the normal state the choroid fills slightly earlier than the retinal circulation. Because of the masking effect of the retinal pigment epithelium the choroidal vessels are not accurately delineated but filling of the choriocapillaris can be observed as a background flush. Frequently the choroid fills in lobular patterns which coalesce after a few seconds into a uniform background (Figure 2.4).

The retinal circulation is outlined more precisely than the choroidal circulation. The angiogram is arbitrarily divided into arterial, capillary, and early, mid and late venous phases, followed by a late recirculatory phase. In practice it must be remembered that the flow is dynamic and continuous; the capillary phase at the disc will be well ahead of the periphery. The exact phasing of abnormalities on angiography is not always important but assessment of whether abnormalities occur early or late during the transit of fluorescein may be significant.

Arterial phase – This is usually 5–10 s after injection, with arterial filling in the retina (the choroid usually fills slightly earlier). During this phase the arteriolar blood column becomes rapidly wider to fill the whole lumen (Figure 2.4a).

Capillary phase – This is often difficult to distinguish precisely from the arterial phase. In young subjects or patients with clear optic media retinal capillaries can be directly visualized (Figure 2.4b).

Early venous phase – The major veins begin to fill around the posterior pole of the eye. Because venous flow is slower and less turbulent than arterial flow, fluorescein tends to fill the veins in a laminar fashion. Dye enters the veins from adjacent small tributaries and remains close to the vein wall (Figure 2.4c).

Mid-venous phase – Arterioles begin to fade and veins fill more. Some laminar flow persists but the veins begin to fill completely (Figure 2.4d).

Late venous phase – Arterioles are now pale and all veins are full (Figure 2.4e).

Late phase – All vessels fade and are equally filled by recirculating fluorescein in the bloodstream (Figure 2.4f). Background choroidal fluorescence also fades.

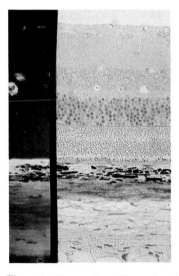

Figure 2.3 Transection of the retina showing confinement of the fluorescein in the lumen of retinal capillaries by the inner blood–retinal barrier and by the retinal pigment epithelium at the outer blood–retinal barrier. (Courtesy of Professor John Marshall)

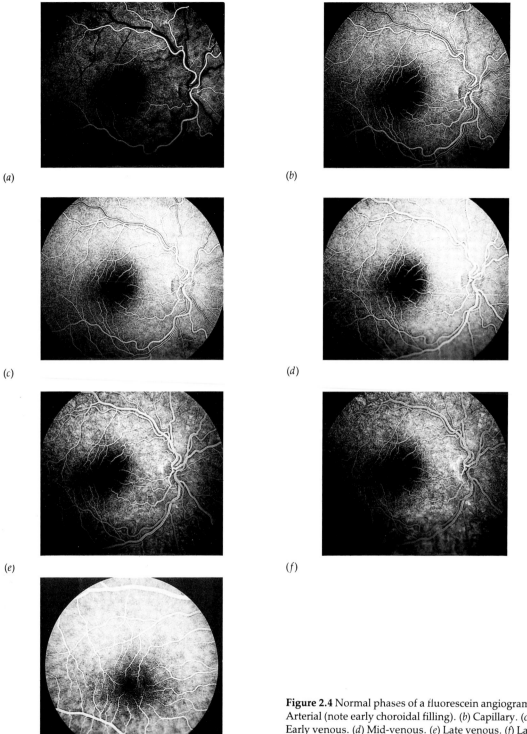

Figure 2.4 Normal phases of a fluorescein angiogram. (*a*) Arterial (note early choroidal filling). (*b*) Capillary. (*c*) Early venous. (*d*) Mid-venous. (*e*) Late venous. (*f*) Late. (*g*) Capillary phase of macula (note perifoveal capillary free zone)

Pseudofluorescence

This occurs if there is overlap in the transmission characteristics of the exciting and barrier filters. Blue light will, therefore, be reflected from the fundus, pass through the barrier filter and expose the camera film. The film will look as if there has been fluorescence whereas there has been merely blue light transmission. The condition is most commonly seen late in the angiogram following reflection of light by large white areas in the fundus.

Autofluorescence

This is seen mainly but not exclusively in drusen of the optic disc. The material in the drusen acts similarly to fluorescein being excited by blue light and emitting green light. The lesions appear fluorescent in the absence of fluorescein (Figure 2.5).

Abnormal angiography

The blood vessels in the retina may demonstrate abnormal filling in several ways: it may be slow, partial or non-existent. The calibre of a vessel may be irregular or the vessel may be either tortuous or abnormally straight. If endothelial cell function is compromised, fluorescein crosses the inner blood–retinal barrier and may stain a vessel wall or leak into the neuroretina, suggesting oedema in an extravascular space (always abnormal as there is no extravascular space in the normal retina). Damage to the pigment epithelium causes loss of the outer blood–retinal barrier with staining of the cells or pooling of fluorescein in the subretinal space or retina.

Hyperfluorescence

Hyperfluorescence denotes an increase in fluorescence compared with a normal angiogram. Although this often means fluorescein is leaking from vessels or pooling abnormally there are some circumstances when this is not the case.

Disorders reducing the amount of pigment in the retinal pigment epithelium will reveal the underlying choroidal circulation. This is known as a transmission defect or 'windowing', i.e. increased visualization of the normal choriocapillaris. This type of hyperfluorescence fades as the dye transit progresses into the late phase, in contrast to hyperfluorescence from leakage which increases in the late stages of the angiogram.

Hypofluorescence

Hypofluorescence denotes a deceased amount of fluorescence compared with a normal angiogram. It may follow closure of vessels but may also result from areas of masking by pigments, which absorb

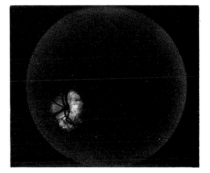

(a)

(b)

Figure 2.5 Autofluorescence of (a) optic disc drusen and (b) macular deposits

all the excitatory blue light. Both blood and melanin cause marked hypofluorescence of the underlying tissues. Exudates and cotton wool spots cause minimal masking of normal fluorescence.

Abnormal angiography of specific conditions will be considered in detail in the subsequent chapters but it should be remembered that retinal blood vessels have a limited range of responses to disease processes. Similar angiographic appearances may, therefore, result from different underlying causes.

Further reading

DUANE, T. D. Fluorescein angiography. In *Clinical Ophthalmology*, Vol. III, Chapter 4, Harper and Row, New York

DUANE, T. D. Fluorescein angiography. In *Clinical Ophthalmology*, Vol. IV, Chapter 33, Harper and Row, New York

KRILL, A. E. (1972) *Hereditary Retinal and Choroidal Diseases*, Vol. I, Harper and Row, New York

RYAN, S. J. (1989) *Retina*, Vol. II, Chapter 57, C. V. Mosby, New York

WISE, G. N., DOLLEY, C. T. and HENKIND, P. (1971) *The Retinal Circulation*, Harper and Row, New York

3

The vascular response to disease and photocoagulation

Vascular response to disease

Regardless of the underlying mechanism inducing vascular damage blood vessels can respond in only a limited number of ways. The major vessels of the retina and choroid may either lose their normal configuration, occlude or, unusually, rupture. The capillary bed similarly may become occluded or become incompetent and extravasate the normal intravascular components into the tissues. Broadly, the effects of retinal vascular disease can be considered to be the result of the primary disorder and the subsequent exudative or ischaemic response, or combinations of both.

Exudative response

Exudation results from loss of blood–retinal barrier (inner or outer) and is manifested by accumulation of plasma fluid and lipid within the neuroretina (Figure 3.1). Localized lesions may give rise to circinate exudation with a ring of exudate surrounding a central vascular defect. Function is lost in those areas of chronic oedema and exudate accumulation and, if the fovea is affected, visual acuity will be reduced. Sometimes exudation may lead to the formation of subretinal fluid and retinal detachment.

Ischaemic response

Ischaemia follows closure of retinal capillaries and leads to retinal hypoxia. Ophthalmoscopically, acute ischaemia of the retina can be suspected by the presence of diffuse sheet-like haemorrhages and cotton wool spots. The latter are accumulations of axoplasmic material which build up on either side of a microinfarct and denote localized damage in the axons of the ganglion cells (Figure 3.2). Signs that may denote longstanding retinal

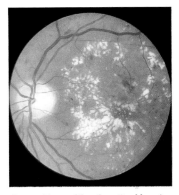

Figure 3.1 Loss of inner blood–retinal barrier with exudates and oedema of the neuroretina

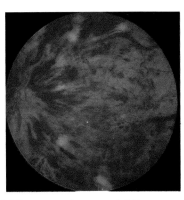

Figure 3.2 Cotton wool spots and diffuse haemorrhage denoting retinal ischaemia

ischaemia include venous beading, venous loops and vessel sheathing.

Hypoxia from under-perfusion of the neuroretina leads to release of one or more factors which induce neovascularization. These neovascular factors act on viable endothelial cells in the retinal circulation and cause proliferation and formation of buds. The buds penetrate the basement membrane of the retinal capillaries, canalize and then migrate through the internal limiting lamina of the retina to lie on the vitreoretinal interface. Subsequently fibrous tissue is laid down around the endothelial cell channels leading to fibrovascular bands. Common sites for neovascularization to occur are the optic disc head, the major arcades of the retina and the surface of the iris. Disorders causing peripheral retinal ischaemia, e.g. S-C disease or retinopathy of prematurity, tend to cause neovascularization in the peripheral or equatorial regions of the retina. Conditions that induce complete anoxia rather than hypoxia of the neuroretina rarely lead to neovascularization because viable endothelial cells are required for induction of the neovascular process. Experimentally and clinically there is evidence that the vitreous and the retinal pigment epithelium have inhibitory properties against neovascularization. New vessel formation is probably a result of an imbalance between stimulatory and inhibitory factors in the retina and adjacent tissues. In view of the serious complications of preretinal neovascularization (vitreous haemorrhage, traction retinal detachment and neovascular glaucoma), reversal of the process should be vigorously pursued by photocoagulation, cryotherapy or, in some cases, vitreoretinal surgery.

Diagnosis of retinal vascular disorders is based on pattern recognition of the basic vessel changes of the primary disease and the subsequent retinal response (exudative, ischaemic or mixed). In most patients the diagnosis is straightforward but in doubtful cases fluorescein angiography may be helpful in establishing the diagnosis and assessing the degree of exudation or ischaemia.

Principles of photocoagulation

The aim of treatment of retinal vascular disorders is to reverse the sight-threatening consequences of

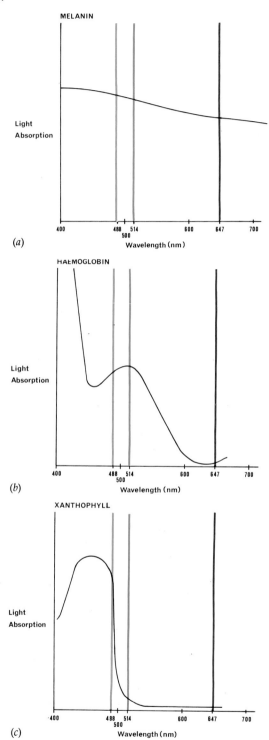

Figure 3.3 Absorption characteristics of ocular pigments. (*a*) Melanin. (*b*) Haemoglobin. (*c*) Xanthophyll

the primary vascular pathology and the subsequent secondary effects. In some conditions (e.g. systemic hypertension) treatment of the primary condition leads to reversal of the vascular abnormalities and specific ocular treatment is not required. For those conditions in which the secondary effects are the predominant cause of visual loss and in whom treatment of the primary disorder is not possible or ineffective (e.g. diabetes) xenon or laser photocoagulation should be considered. During photocoagulation light energy is absorbed by ocular pigments and converted into heat producing a thermal, destructive burn in the cells containing the pigment. If the energy level is high enough there will be additional secondary damage to adjacent tissues which may not themselves contain absorbing pigment. The pigments within the eye capable of absorbing visible light are melanin, haemoglobin, photoreceptor pigments and the luteal pigment, xanthophyll (Figure 3.3).

Photocoagulation can be carried out using a variety of wavelengths of visible light but the site of energy uptake varies with the absorption characteristics of the pigment and the wavelength used. The commonly available lasers are argon, emitting a combination of 70% blue light (488 nm) and 30% green (514 nm); or krypton, emitting red light (647 nm). In the future it is likely that additional dye lasers employing a variety of wavelengths will be available with the capacity to select different emissions depending on therapeutic requirements.

Melanin is an efficient absorber of all wavelengths, particularly for blue light and, therefore, the retinal pigment epithelium and choroid are the major tissues affected by photocoagulation. Haemoglobin does not absorb red light and, therefore, krypton laser energy does not affect blood vessels directly. Blue–green argon laser light is taken up readily by haemoglobin in retinal vessels, a useful property when treating retinal vascular abnormalities. The luteal pigment absorbs blue light efficiently but most green light and nearly all red light is transmitted. Thus photocoagulation around the fovea is less likely to cause xanthophyll uptake and neuroretinal damage if blue light is avoided.

Table 3.1 summarizes the main advantages and disadvantages of the different wavelengths.

Although laser treatment has been used mainly in recent years, photocoagulation can also be administered by a xenon arc. This generates a high-energy, non-coherent white light beam which is absorbed by the retinal pigment epithelium. Compared with laser treatment the burns are larger (2–6°) and tend to be more intense with greater inner retinal destruction (Figure 3.4). Xenon treatment usually leads to greater side-effects such as reduced colour sensation and visual field loss.

Table 3.1 Advantages and disadvantages of different wavelengths

Wavelength	Advantages	Disadvantages
Blue	Well absorbed in RPE (melanin) Well absorbed by haemoglobin: (a) retinal vascular anomalies (b) staunching a bleeding vessel	Uptake by xanthophyll near fovea Power attenuated by: (a) nuclear sclerosis (b) vitreous haemorrhage Possible blue light hazard to photoreceptors
Green	As per blue but poorly absorbed by zanthophyll and safer near fovea	Only 30% of argon output, therefore laser runs at high power
Red	Not absorbed by haemoglobin, therefore: (a) can be used in presence of mild vitreous haemorrhage (b) no retinal vascular damage Less attenuated by nuclear sclerosis More penetrant into choroid than blue/green Not absorbed by xanthophyll	Will not staunch bleeding vessel Choroidal haemorrhages occur close to levels of energy needed for therapeutic effect

Treatment of exudative response

The purpose of treatment is to re-establish a competent blood–retinal barrier. If this can be achieved, retinal oedema and exudate will resolve although the latter can take many months to disappear. Two methods of treatment can be applied:

1. Direct, in which the laser is focused on the abnormality.
2. A grid pattern for diffuse capillary leakage at the macula when no identifiable localized abnormalities are found.

Direct treatment employs blue–green or green laser wavelengths using small applications (100 μm) of brief exposure (0.1 s) with sufficient power to produce slight change within the vascular lesion, i.e. mild blanching of the vessel wall or darkening of the blood within the lumen.

The blue or green light is absorbed by haemoglobin as well as melanin and, therefore, part of the energy is taken up within the microvascular abnormality as well as the retinal pigment epithelium.

Grid pattern treatment involves larger applications (200 μm) of lower power to induce mild blanching of the retinal pigment epithelium. The blood–retinal barrier may be restored but the mechanism whereby this is achieved is not understood; possibly oedema resolves by increased fluid transfer across the pigment epithelium or alternatively there may be some biochemical factor generated which affects endothelial cell function. Any wavelength of the visible spectrum can be used because melanin absorbs efficiently across the spectrum from blue to red. This technique has been used particularly for diabetic macular oedema with few visible vessel changes, or alternatively, following failed direct treatment.

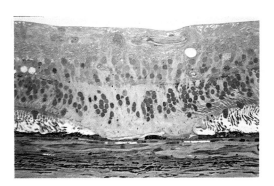

(a)

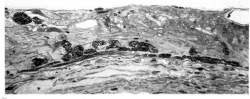

(b)

Figure 3.4 (*a*) Histology of argon laser photocoagulation showing disruption of the retinal pigment epithelium and overlying receptor outer segments. There is mild disorganization of the outer nuclear layer but sparing of the inner retinal layers. (*b*) Histology of xenon photocoagulation showing disruption of all layers of the neuroretina with pigment clumping and migration into the neuroretina. (Courtesy of Professor J. Marshall)

Treatment of the ischaemic response

The principle of photocoagulation of ischaemic retina differs from the exudative response and an indirect method is used. The laser burns are applied to areas of the peripheral fundus which are under-perfused. On most occasions brief (0.1 s), large (500 μm) applications of a power just sufficient to produce blanching of the retinal pigment epithelium are used; there is no evidence that intense burns are more effective than mild burns and the former produce greater side-effects. The treatment is scattered over the ischaemic retina, avoiding the major retinal blood vessels, and is described as scatter or panretinal photocoagulation.

The mechanism of how indirect treatment works is ill-understood but is presumed to reverse the imbalance between the factors which stimulate or inhibit endothelial cell proliferation. Destruction of the pigment epithelium may reduce the production of neovascular factor from the neuroretina by altering the haemodynamics of the retinal circulation or by reducing retinal hypoxia. Pigment epithelial burns also allow greater retinal oxygenation from the choroidal circulation. Alternatively photocoagulation may lead to more rapid egress of the neovascular factor from the eye through the altered pigment epithelium, reducing the stimulus for neovascularization.

Scatter retinal photocoagulation is highly effective in reversing active neovascularization in diabetic retinopathy and should be considered as a possible treatment option in proliferative vascular retinopathy of any cause. Inactive fibrous proliferative retinopathy will not be reversed by photocoagulation and treatment is usually contraindicated in such cases because it may induce retinal traction which may lead to retinal detachment.

Adverse reactions

In common with many modern therapies photocoagulation produces adverse reactions. These can be considered as either side-effects which may be expected to occur in nearly all treated patients or complications which occur rarely and result from mishap.

The side-effects of photocoagulation are a consequence of the tissue destruction produced by treatment. Patients will nearly always experience such effects to some degree and should be warned of them prior to commencing treatment. Dazzling and transient myopia are common and soon pass off but after heavy treatment may take a few days to do so. Pigment epithelial and photoreceptor destruction lead to alterations in colour perception, nyctalopia and to loss of visual field. This is common after extensive panretinal photocoagulation and may occasionally have serious implications for patients' welfare, such as inability to hold a driving licence owing to peripheral field constriction. Photocoagulation around the macula may cause noticeable paracentral scotomata which can interfere with reading, particularly if the fellow eye has poor acuity.

Complications of photocoagulation are uncommon, particularly when care is exercised and treatment is carried out by an experienced operator. Complications arise from either laser energy being misdirected and absorbed inappropriately or by adverse consequences of correctly placed treatment.

Poor focusing of the laser can lead to energy uptake in the cornea or lens, particularly when nuclear sclerosis is present. Fortunately resolution of corneal or lenticular burns is usually complete. Inability to define the fovea may lead to direct foveal damage and loss of central vision. This is particularly likely when treating macular subretinal new vessels because the fovea can be difficult to identify.

Complications from treatment which has been correctly placed include retinal, subretinal or choroidal haemorrhage from vessel rupture, traction retinal detachment from fibrous tissue contraction, and neuroretinal damage from xanthophyll uptake. Rarer consquences of laser treatment are subretinal new vessel membrane formation at the macula, and angle closure glaucoma from heavy peripheral retinal photocoagulation which can induce shallowing of the anterior chamber from choroidal effusion.

In the majority of patients adverse reactions are not a long-term problem but the benefits of treatment always have to be considered against the possibility of side-effects. When vision is threatened seriously, as in proliferative diabetic retinopathy, photocoagulation should not be withheld on the grounds of some risk to field constriction. For self-limiting disorders such as central serous retinopathy careful consideration should be given prior to treatment.

Further reading

ARCHER, D. B. (1977) Intraretinal, preretinal and subretinal new vessels. *Transactions of the Ophthalmic Society of the UK*, **97**, 449–456.

BOULTON, M. E., MCLEOD, D. and GARNER, A. (1988) Vasoproliferative retinopathies; clinical, morphogenetic and modulatory aspects. *Eye*, **2**, (suppl.), 5124–5139

HANSCOM, T. A. (1982) Indirect treatment of peripheral retinal neovascularisation. *American Journal of Ophthalmology*, **93**, 88–91

KISSUN, R. D., HILL, C. R., GARNER, A., PHILLIPS, J. B., KUMAR, S. and WEISS, J. B. (1982) A low-molecular-weight angiogenic factor in cat retina. *British Journal of Ophthalmology*, **66**, 165–169

L'ESPERENCE, F. A. (1989) *Ophthalmic Lasers*, Vols. I and II, C. V. Mosby, New York

MCLEOD, D., MARSHALL, J., KOHNER, E. M. and BIRD, A. C. (1977) The role of axoplasmic transport in the pathogenesis of retinal cotton-wool spots. *British Journal of Ophthalmology*, **61**, 177-191

MCLEOD, D., MARSHALL, J. and KOHNER, E. M. (1980) Role of axoplasmic transport in the pathophysiology of ischaemic disc swelling. *British Journal of Ophthalmology*, **64**, 247–261

MARSHALL, J. and BIRD, A. C. (1979) A comparative histopathological study of argon and krypton laser irradiations of the human retina. *British Journal of Ophthalmology*, **63**, 657–668

MICHAELSON, I. C. (1980) *Textbook of the Fundus of the Eye*, 3rd edn., Churchill Livingstone, London

PATZ, A. (1982) Clinical and experimental studies on retinal neovascularization. *American Journal of Ophthalmology*, **94**, 715–743

RYAN, S. J. (1989) *Retina*, Vol. II, Chapters 58–62, C. V. Mosby, New York

SPENCER, W. H. (1985) *Ophthalmic Pathology*, Vol. II, W. B. Saunders and Co., Philadelphia

STEFANSSON, E., HATCHELL, D. L., FISHER, B. L., SUTHERLAND, F. S. and MACHEMER, R. (1986) Panretinal photocoagulation and retinal oxygenation in normal and diabetic cats. *American Journal of Ophthalmology*, **101**, 657–664

WISE, G. N., DOLLEY C. T. and HENKIND, P. (1971) *The Retinal Circulation*, Harper and Row, New York

4

Major vessel occlusion

Central retinal artery occlusion

The central retinal artery is an end artery. Acute obstruction of the blood flow causes immediate, profound disturbance of vision of the affected eye because a collateral circulation cannot develop.

Aetiology

The majority of patients with central retinal artery obstruction are elderly and, therefore, come from the population at risk of arterial occlusive disease. Systemic hypertension, arteriosclerosis, carotid artery disease, diabetes mellitus, giant cell arteritis and ischaemic heart disease have all been associated with central retinal artery obstruction.

Pathogenesis

The central retinal artery becomes obstructed either by vessel wall disease (atheroma, arteritis) or by an embolus formed in the proximal circulation (e.g. in the heart following arrhythmias or carotid artery atheroma).

Regardless of the underlying cause, the effect of retinal artery obstruction is profound ischaemia of the inner layers of the neuroretina with cloudy swelling of the neurons and subsequent atrophy of the inner nuclear and ganglion cell layers.

Clinical features

Patients are aware of unilateral loss of vision beginning either as a shadow or 'brightness' which spreads rapidly across the field of vision over a few minutes.

Ophthalmoscopically the striking feature of acute central retinal artery obstruction is pallor of the fundus from axonal swelling and a 'cherry red spot' at the fovea. Segmentation of the blood column in the retinal arteries and veins may be observed and there is frequently a peripapillary cuff of obstructed white, retrograde axoplasmic flow (Figure 4.1a). The optic disc appears normal because it is supplied by the ciliary circulation, hence the build up of retrograde axoplasmic transport near the disc margin from the viable portion of the axons in the optic nerve.

Three to four weeks after the occlusion the retinal signs resolve leaving an atrophic, thin neuroretina, attenuated retinal vessels and pale optic disc. As a result of severe neuroretinal anoxia it is rare for neovascularization to develop later.

Investigations

Fluorescein angiography in the acute stage shows slowed or complete failure of dye to enter the retinal circulation but the choroid and optic disc fluoresce normally. Retrograde filling of the retinal circulation close to the disc may occur from the

19

capillaries supplied by the circle of Zinn (Figure 4.1b).

Giant cell arteritis must always be considered in the elderly, especially in the presence of a high plasma viscosity or ESR (see p. 22). A source of emboli should be searched for by carotid artery auscultation, carotid ultrasound and where indicated angiography. A cardiac examination should also be performed and diabetes, systemic hypertension or generalized arteriopathy excluded.

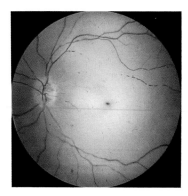

(a)

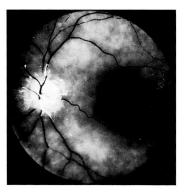

(b)

Figure 4.1 (a) Acute central retinal artery occlusion – note peripapillary axoplasmic block and cloudy swelling of ganglion cell axons. (b) Angiogram of (a) with obstructed retinal artery but disc filling from circle of Zinn

Treatment

Because neuronal damage occurs within minutes of occlusion no treatment has been found to have universal benefit. A variety of treatments have been attempted with occasional success and, therefore, should be tried in hope rather than expectation of improvement. Rebreathing into a paper bag to induce hypercapnoeic vasodilatation, or lowering of intraocular pressure by ocular massage, acetozolamide and paracentesis to dislodge emboli can be tried. Long-term vasodilator drugs are ineffective but low-dose aspirin treatment or anticoagulation may help to prevent further embolization.

If carotid artery or cardiac disease is identified appropriate specialist attention should be sought, especially if carotid stenosis is present requiring endarterectomy. Prophylactic treatment with systemic steroids must be given in cases of giant cell arteritis to prevent occlusion in the fellow eye.

Transient ischaemic attacks

These produce episodic loss of vision in part or all of the visual field. Patients usually describe a cloud or curtain advancing across the vision which then recedes some minutes later.

Fundus examination can be normal but there may be emboli visible in the retinal arterioles or small retinal haemorrhages present from capillary obstruction.

Such patients frequently have an identifiable source of emboli and this should be diligently sought for in order to prevent later complete retinal artery obstruction or cerebrovascular infarction. Low-dose aspirin treatment should be instigated, as for carotid disease.

Transient ischaemic attacks in the vertebrobasilar circulation produce episodic homonymous hemianopia and patients may confuse this with visual disturbance in the eye on the side of the hemianopia. There are no fundus signs but investigation and treatment is on similar lines to carotid artery disease. Migraine is a common cause of transient visual loss but careful questioning into family history or associated symptoms usually provides the diagnosis and may save much time and anxiety spent in undertaking investigations.

Ciliary artery occlusion

Aetiology

The causes of ciliary artery obstruction are similar to those of central retinal artery occlusion but embolization is less frequently found whereas hypertension and arteriosclerosis are more common.

Clinical features

Optic nerve – The most frequent manifestation of ciliary artery obstruction is sudden severe loss of vision from infarction of the optic nerve head, known as anterior ischaemic optic neuropathy. Closure of vessels supplying the circle of Zinn results in axonal swelling at the optic disc from interruption of axoplasmic flow.

Ophthalmoscopically the optic disc is swollen and frequently has splinter haemorrhages in the axonal layer and around the disc margin. There is obstruction of orthograde axoplasmic flow visible around the disc margins but the peripheral retina and macula appear normal (Figure 4.2).

In common with central retinal artery obstruction recovery is usually limited and a few weeks after the occlusive episode the optic disc is pale and the neuroretina atrophic.

Segmental obstruction – Owing to the anastomotic arrangement of the ciliary arteries supplying the circle of Zinn obstruction of a ciliary artery sometimes leads to segmental optic nerve head infarction and arcuate field defects; the size of the field defect depending on the extent of the infarct.

Swelling, then subsequent atrophy of a sector of the optic nerve, can be observed.

Peripheral ciliary artery obstruction is rare and does not usually cause significant visual disturbance. Anastomotic channels allow a collateral circulation to become established which prevents outer retinal ischaemia.

Acute infarction is rarely observed. It produces patchy whitening of the retinal pigment epithelium and sometimes an associated serous detachment of the neuroretina.

Old peripheral choroidal infarcts show as sectorial areas of pigment epithelial atrophy and clumping of melanin (Figure 4.3).

Investigations

Fluorescein angiography is not always helpful in the diagnosis of ciliary artery occlusion as the choroidal circulation is less visible than the retinal circulation and often fills normally. Sometimes sectors of the choroid can be observed to fill slowly or incompletely around the optic disc in cases of anterior ischaemic optic neuropathy, suggesting occlusion of one or more short ciliary arteries.

Blood and systemic circulation investigations should be carried out in a similar way to cases of retinal artery occlusion.

Treatment

Treatment is ineffective in restoring vision following optic nerve head infarction. The methods used for retinal artery obstruction may be tried but

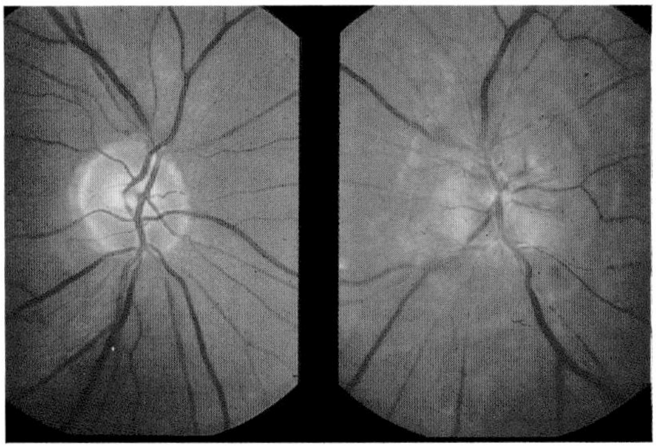

Figure 4.2 Left anterior ischaemic optic neuropathy

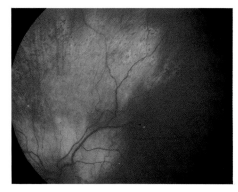

Figure 4.3 Peripheral old choroidal infarction

measures to reduce intra-ocular pressure are unlikely to succeed. Systemic steroids have been tried to reduce swelling within the optic disc to alleviate compression but there is little evidence of success. Prophylactic treatment with systemic steroids should be given in cases of giant cell arteritis to prevent infarction in the fellow eye.

Giant cell arteritis must be considered in all cases of either central retinal artery occlusion or anterior ischaemic optic neuropathy in the elderly. The disease causes an inflammatory reaction within medium sized arteries, producing infiltration of the vessel wall and obstruction of the lumen. Only vessels possessing an internal elastic lamina are involved and the vessel becomes infiltrated with lymphocytes, plasma cells and giant cells.

The patients affected are aged over 60 and usually over 70 years of age. Symptoms include muscle and joint pains, malaise, weight loss, jaw aching on chewing, temporal pains in the head and visual loss. There is also a risk of cardiac and cerebral vascular occlusion. The ESR and plasma viscosity are very high in almost all cases and these should be used as confirmatory tests. A biopsy of an affected portion of a temporal artery can be taken to obtain histological proof of the diagnosis but it is frequently not necessary and should not give rise to delay in treatment. Biopsy may be helpful in cases where the history or ESR are equivocal.

The importance of identifying giant cell arteritis lies in the high risk of occlusion in the fellow eye. Once the diagnosis is established the patient should be treated with high-dose systemic corticosteroids until the ESR falls. When a response is obtained the steroid dosage can be reduced and then titrated against the ESR. A small dose of steroid may be necessary for 2 years or more but eventually the disease becomes inactive and treatment can be stopped.

Branch retinal and cilioretinal arteriolar occlusions

Branch retinal arterioles

These have a different structure from the central retinal artery (see Chapter 1) and are, therefore, not subject to the same risk of arteriosclerotic or atheromatous occlusion. However, not infrequently emboli impact in the peripheral retinal arterioles and may cause central or peripheral visual field loss from ischaemia in the affected sector of the retina. On rare occasions an inflammatory focus in the retina (e.g. acute toxoplasmosis) may obstruct an adjacent retinal arteriole.

Clinical features – Not all emboli produce visual symptoms but when axonal damage is extensive or occurs near the macula patients become aware of visual field loss, particularly when close to fixation.

Ophthalmoscopically acute embolic infarction produces a sector of retinal pallor typical of cloudy swelling. The sector is based on the vascular territory peripheral to the site of occlusion and, if the embolus is still present, it is nearly always lodged in an arteriolar division, where the vessel lumen becomes reduced in cross-section (Figure 4.4). In some cases the embolus has become lysed

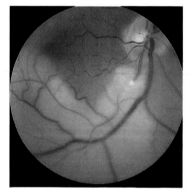

(*a*)

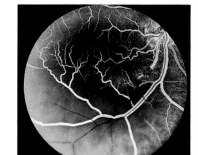

(*b*)

Figure 4.4 (*a*) Retinal arteriolar embolus and infarction. (*b*) Angiogram of (*a*); note retrograde filling of distal portion of arteriole

and is no longer visible in the fundus but in others multiple emboli can be seen. After resolution of the acute signs the affected arteriole appears narrowed and sheathed or may be reduced to a thin white thread.

Investigation and treatment is the same as for central retinal arteriolar embolization. The source of emboli should be identified and, if possible, removed. Aspirin should be given in a low dose to reduce the risk of further ischaemic attacks.

Cilioretinal arteriolar obstruction

This produces cloudy swelling and infarction in a circumscribed area of the retina similar to the appearance of a peripheral retinal arterial occlu-

sion. The affected sector extends from the optic disc and corresponds to the area of supply of the cilioretinal arteriole (Figure 4.5).

Because the affected vessel is derived from the ciliary circulation, obstruction may be caused by any of the conditions leading to ciliary artery obstruction. Cilioretinal or branch retinal arteriolar occlusion is sometimes observed in cases of central retinal vein occlusion. When this occurs the territory of the cilioretinal arteriole shows cloudy swelling and is relatively free of haemorrhages and cotton wool spots, unlike the surrounding areas which have multiple haemorrhages and typical signs of venous occlusion (Figure 4.6).

Microemboli can impact in the retinal circulation in cases of subacute bacterial endocarditis. This produces typical lesions known as Roth's spots with pale centres surrounded by haemorrhage. They are caused by small infected fragments from the heart valves which lodge in the small arterioles of the retinal circulation. They are usually too small to cause large areas of retinal infarction (Figure 4.7).

Central retinal vein occlusion

Obstruction of a central retinal vein is one of the most common causes of acute visual loss.

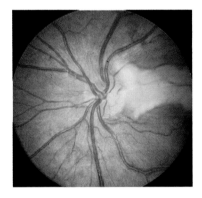

(*a*)

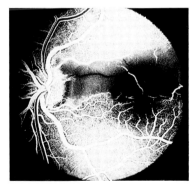

(*b*)

Figure 4.5 (*a*) Cilioretinal arteriolar obstruction – note axoplasmic block where nerve fibres cross into ischaemic area. (*b*) Angiogram of (*a*) with absent arterial filling

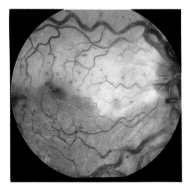

Figure 4.6 Cilioretinal arteriolar obstruction following central retinal vein occlusion

Pathogenesis

The development of central vein occlusion follows a number of pathological disorders but in a large proportion of cases there is no obvious cause. Not only is the origin frequently unknown but complete occlusion of the vein may not have taken place in all cases. Serial histological examination of occluded veins has sometimes demonstrated no physical obstruction of the vessel lumen.

An association with central retinal vein occlusion has been found in patients with systemic hypertension, hyperviscosity syndromes, raised intra-ocular pressure and compressive lesions of the anterior optic nerve and has also been reported in pregnancy and woman taking oral contraceptives.

In common with nearly all vascular disorders central vein occlusion is mainly a disease of the elderly. It was thought that concomitant retinal artery disease was necessary for vein occlusion to occur and there has been some experimental evidence to support this. Although generalized arteriosclerotic disease may be present in some patients with central vein occlusion, obstruction can also occur in young patients and those with plasma hyperviscosity in the absence of arterial

disease. Hypergammaglobulinaemia, multiple myeloma, polycythaemia (primary or secondary) and chronic leukaemias may also be associated with vein obstruction.

Venous occlusion associated with raised intra-ocular pressure is well recognized. The fact that occlusion may occur in the presence of high intra-ocular pressure without pathological cupping of the disc would suggest that the pressure rise *per se* rather than distortion of the lamina cribrosa is the important factor in such cases.

A further feature in the development of venous occlusion is the role of posture and sleep. Central venous pressure in the head increases on lying down, thus increasing the retinal and choroidal venous pressure and impairing blood flow from the eye. Intra-ocular pressure rises briefly on lying down but usually falls rapidly to normal. There is evidence to suggest that there is a reduced capacity for the intra-ocular pressure to readjust in patients with retinal vein occlusion, which may account for the obstruction so often occurring overnight.

Clinical features

Patients with central vein occlusion experience acute loss of vision but the degree of visual disturbance can be variable. Some patients are hardly aware of any deficit whereas others have almost total loss of vision. Unlike arterial occlusions which occur at any time of day, patients with central vein occlusions are usually aware of blurred vision on waking in the morning.

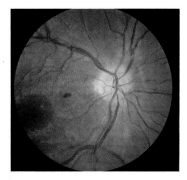

Figure 4.7 Roth's spot in a case of subacute bacterial endocarditis

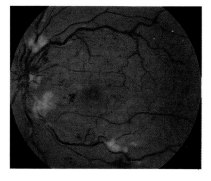

Figure 4.8 Central retinal vein occlusion

The fundus picture of acute vein occlusion is often characteristic, with multiple haemorrhages throughout the retina, a swollen optic disc and

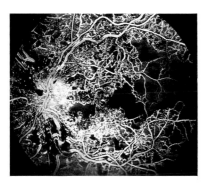

(a)

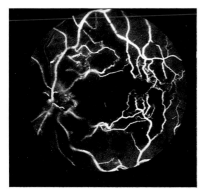

(b)

(c)

Figure 4.9 Angiograms of central vein occlusion. (a) No capillary occlusion. (b) Partial capillary occlusion. (c) Severe capillary occlusion

dilated tortuous veins (Figure 4.8). Cotton wool spots may be present. In some mild occlusions the appearance can be deceptive with minimal macular oedema and a few scattered haemorrhages, particularly around the equator. In such cases fluorescein angiography can be helpful in revealing more extensive capillary changes than are readily apparent on ophthalmoscopy.

Disc swelling and venous engorgement resolve over a period of a few weeks but often many months are required for retinal haemorrhages to clear. The final appearance after resolution of the acute phase varies with the degree of damage to the capillary bed. In mild cases it can sometimes be difficult to detect any abnormality and visual acuity can be nearly normal, but most patients have some long-term visual loss and the macula may have persistent cystoid oedema or atrophic changes of the pigment epithelium. In more severe cases the peripheral arteries and veins are narrowed and frequently sheathed. The neuroretina may be thinned where ischaemia is present; small vessel tortuosity and scattered haemorrhages are common findings. The disc is often atrophic and may demonstrate tortuous collateral channels.

Previously, central vein occlusion was divided into two sub-groups: partial and complete. This was dependent on whether the retina demonstrated mild vascular damage with a mainly exudative response or whether there was more severe capillary loss and ischaemia. It is now recognized that the degree of capillary disruption varies from case to case ranging from dilatation without loss at one extreme through mild closure to severe closure at the other extreme (Figure 4.9).

Although the distinction between partial and complete occlusion is not very useful, about 10% of patients present with a mild occlusive episode and some weeks or months later have a second attack with severe capillary loss. Interestingly, capillary closure has been shown experimentally to continue for a week after occlusion has occurred.

Investigations

Fluorescein angiography is necessary in order to assess the degree of retinal capillary closure because the ophthalmoscopic appearance can sometimes be deceptive. When extensive ischaemia is present there is a significant risk of later development of rubeosis iridis and subsequent neovascular glaucoma. This dreaded complication should be avoided whenever possible and angiography is helpful in assessing the risk of rubeosis iridis. Angiography should be carried out approximately 1 month after occlusion or sooner if the haemorrhages allow visualization of the capillary bed over a reasonable area of the fundus. When multiple cotton wool spots are present the likelihood of ischaemia is greater but, because they are transient, allowance should not be placed on the presence of cotton wool spots to diagnose ischaemia.

Intra-ocular pressure should be measured in both eyes. Immediately after central vein occlusion ocular pressure usually falls and may be normal. The true aetiology of the occlusion may, therefore, be missed if the pressure in the fellow eye is not measured.

Blood pressure and haematological investigation should be undertaken to exclude any systemic cause such as hyperviscosity states. The possibility of such conditions is greater when the occlusion takes place in younger patients but a number of patients in the third and fourth decades suffer a typical central vein occlusion in the absence of any identifiable cause. This condition used to be termed vasculitis but this is incorrect as there is no inflammatory process present. It is possible, however, for an inflammatory lesion or tumour within the optic nerve head to lead to subsequent vein occlusion.

Treatment

Treatment of central vein occlusion is aimed mainly at preventing neovascular glaucoma (see below) and little can be done to restore diminished vision. If ocular hypertension or glaucoma is present the intra-ocular pressure must be lowered especially to reduce the risk to the fellow eye.

Grid pattern laser photocoagulation has been tried in cases of persistent macular oedema. Some success has been shown in reducing retinal oedema but the long-term visual outcome in such patients is not known. No drug treatment is of proven benefit.

Neovascular glaucoma

Rubeosis iridis and subsequent neovascular glaucoma occurs in approximately 25% of patients suffering a central vein occlusion. When retinal capillary dilatation without closure is present the risk of rubeosis iridis is non-existent. In cases in which the area of closure is considerable the risk of rubeosis increases and when total capillary loss is present the risk of rubeosis is nearly 80%. Unlike diabetic patients, in whom the proliferative neovascular process usually starts in the fundus, in central retinal vein occlusion the response is on the iris surface and over the drainage angle causing intractable blockage of aqueous drainage. The difference in the response between diabetes and vein occlusion may be explained by the lack of viable endothelial cells in the retina following severe central retinal vein occlusion, thus preventing retinal or optic disc new vessel formation, but permeation of neovascular factors into the anterior chamber does not prevent iris neovascularization. On some occasions optic disc or retinal neovascularization can follow central vein occlusion but in such cases retinal capillary closure is only partial allowing viable endothelial cells to survive and proliferate.

The onset of glaucoma occurs approximately 3 months after central vein occlusion but may occur as quickly as 2 weeks or as late as 6 months. The features are a red tender, painful eye with corneal oedema, iris rubeosis and severely elevated intra-ocular pessure. As the condition is largely preventable prophylactic treatment should be carried out on all cases at risk, i.e. those with marked retinal ischaemia. Panretinal photocoagulation usually prevents the development of rubeosis and often reverses early rubeosis. Treatment should, therefore, be tried in such early cases and a response is usually obtained with 1500 applications (see p. 16).

Once glaucoma is established treatment with atropine and steroid drops should be tried to alleviate the pain. In some cases retrobulbar alcohol injections or enucleation are necessary.

Branch retinal vein occlusion

Obstruction of branch retinal veins is a common clinical occurrence. The occlusion may affect a hemisphere, a quadrant, a macular or a peripheral vein but temporal veins (especially superior) are more commonly affected than nasal veins.

Aetiology

Occlusion of a branch retinal vein occurs at an arterio-venous crossing, where arteriole and vein share a common adventitial sheath. Conditions that cause arteriolar thickening lead to compression of the vein and subsequent obstruction. Branch vein occlusion is the commonest reason for patients with systemic hypertension to present to ophthalmologists.

Clinical features

When veins draining the macular area are affected patients are aware of blurred vision. The degree of blurring is variable and unlike patients with central vein occlusion the visual loss is not necessarily proportional to the amount of capillary closure. A more important factor seems to be the state of the surviving capillaries around the fovea and there is a better prognosis for vision if the perifoveal arcade is intact.

The ophthalmoscopic appearance is similar to central retinal vein occlusion, but only the territory drained by the affected vein is involved (Figure 4.10a). At the point of the occlusion at the arterio-venous crossing the proximal portion of the vein is narrowed and the distal portion is dilated. Multiple retinal haemorrhages are present and cotton wool spots frequently found. As the acute signs resolve over several weeks the cotton wool spots and haemorrhages absorb leaving retinal oedema, dilated tortuous capillaries and, sometimes, exudates. At the borders of the territory of the occluded vein with neighbouring healthy veins dilated collateral channels are often observed. In some cases the retinal circulation becomes re-established with good functional recovery.

Investigations

Fluorescein angiography is strongly recommended to establish the state of the surviving capillaries and the degree of retinal ischaemia in the occluded territory, particularly with larger occlusions. It is best carried out after 2 or 3 months allowing many of the retinal haemorrhages to absorb, thereby reducing masking. Macular oedema is often present but may resolve after some months. In cases in which the perifoveal capillary arcade is intact the prognosis for visual recovery is better than in those cases in which the arcade is disrupted. When a quadrant or hemisphere vein is occluded and there is extensive capillary closure, neovascularization may develop at the optic disc

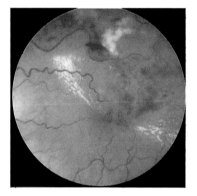

(a)

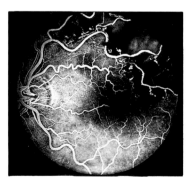

(b)

Figure 4.10 (*a*) Upper temporal branch vein occlusion. (*b*) Angiogram of (*a*). Note intact perifoveal arcade. Acuity was 6/9 in spite of extensive ischaemia

or peripheral retina (Figure 4.11). Photocoagulation may, therefore, be required to regress new vessels and reduce the risk of vitreous haemorrhage (see below).

Blood pressure measurements and haematological investigations for hyperviscosity syndromes should be instigated. Unlike central vein occlusions there is no association between branch retinal vein occlusion and raised intra-ocular pressure unless a hemisphere vein is involved on the optic disc.

Treatment

Reports on the treatment of macular oedema from branch vein occlusion by photocoagulation have been contradictory. Macular oedema can be resolved in many cases but, in some, the oedema will resolve spontaneously after several months. Moreover resolution of macular oedema does not necessarily improve visual acuity although further

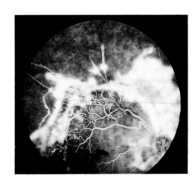

(a)

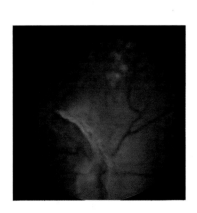

(b)

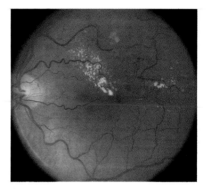

(a)

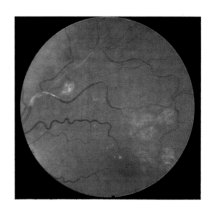

(b)

(c)

Figure 4.11 (a) Disc neovascularization following branch vein occlusion 18 months previously. (b) Angiogram of (a) showing extensive capillary closure. (c) Regression of new vessels after laser treatment

Figure 4.12 (a) Same case as Figure 4.10. Increase in parafoveal exudate deposit at fovea. (b) 1 year after treatment. Note exudate resolution and vessel sheathing from longstanding vein occlusion

deterioration is usually prevented. It would seem reasonable, therefore, to treat those patients in whom the visual acuity can be shown to be falling over a period of months, by direct photocoagulation of the visible vascular abnormalities. When increasing exudate deposition at the macula is observed laser treatment should be given to prevent further loss of central vision (Figure 4.12).

Proliferative retinopathy

Proliferative retinopathy follows in those cases of branch vein occlusion with extensive capillary loss (Figure 4.11). Unlike central vein occlusion rubeosis iridis is not a complication but optic disc or retinal neovascularization is found in 20–30% of cases following branch vein occlusion of a quadrant or greater, in which there is extensive ischaemia.

As the development of neovascularization occurs between 1 and 3 years after the venous occlusion, patients with retinal ischaemia shown by angiography should be followed for a prolonged period. If new vessels have not developed after 3 years, observation can usually be discontinued.

Once neovascularization has occurred there is a considerable risk of vitreous haemorrhage and severe loss of vision. Because many eyes with ischaemic branch vein occlusion have good acuity, vitreous haemorrhage can be very disturbing to the patient and may require vitrectomy. Neovascularization therefore should be treated by scatter photocoagulation to the area of the ischaemic retina because the active proliferation responds well to treatment.

Peripheral ischaemic branch vein occlusions, which do not affect visual acuity, may remain unnoticed until bleeding occurs from neovascularization. Venous occlusion should be considered in the differential diagnosis of sudden vitreous haemorrhage, particularly in patients with a history of hypertension.

Vortex vein occlusion

Owing to the extensive anastomotic bed of the choriocapillaris, occlusion of a single vortex vein does not lead to a disturbance of vision or fundus abnormality. On those occasions when multiple vortex vein obstructions occur the fundus shows choroidal effusion with or without secondary retinal detachment. The two clinical conditions in which vortex vein obstruction is encountered are (1) following retinal detachment surgery and (2) in the uveal effusion syndrome.

Retinal detachment surgery

This may lead to serous effusion in the choroid (Figure 4.13). Most commonly but not invariably it follows an encircling procedure when the silicone explant lies behind the equator of the eye and therefore care must be taken not to place explants too posteriorly. Encircling bands at the equator or anteriorly are usually not complicated by choroidal effusion but extensive use of broad tyres may impair vortex vein drainage.

It is rare for intervention to be necessary as the effusion usually resolves spontaneously after a few weeks. However, choroidal effusion may be accompanied by shallowing of the anterior chamber and sometimes by secondary angle closure glaucoma. Release of the encircling explant may then be necessary to reduce the choroidal effusion, or alternatively choroidal fluid can be drained.

Uveal effusion syndrome

This rare condition results from chronic vortex vein obstruction leading to persistent peripheral choroidal effusion. Thickening of the sclera causes

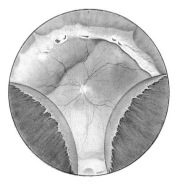

Figure 4.13 Choroidal effusion following retinal detachment surgery. (Reproduced by courtesy of T. Tarrant)

impairment of blood flow in the vortex veins and frequently there is an associated secondary retinal detachment with mobile subretinal fluid. Either sex can be affected and the condition occurs mainly in the fifth to seventh decades of life. Initially symptoms of visual disturbance may be mild as the choroidal effusion is peripheral but once the retina becomes detached loss of visual field becomes apparent. Both choroidal and retinal detachment tend to persist for months or years but spontaneous resolution can follow ultimately. Longstanding choroidal effusion leads to characteristic melanotic mottling of the peripheral retinal pigment epithelium.

Systemic steroids have been advocated for the treatment of uveal effusion syndrome but are ineffective. Better results have been obtained by partial thickness sclerotomies in each quadrant between the recti muscles. This allows the protein rich fluid in the choroidal effusion to percolate through the remaining thinned scleral bed. Postoperatively both choroidal and retinal detachment may take several weeks to resolve.

Similar choroidal effusions have been found in cases of nanophthalmos in which there is gross hypermetropia, a short axial length of the globe and scleral thickening. Surgical procedures in nanophthalmos, particularly glaucoma operations for angle closure, have a high incidence of persistent uveal effusion. Choroidal effusion and secondary retinal detachment may also be seen in cases of posterior scleritis. However, this is usually unilateral and is often associated with ocular pain and mild proptosis.

Further reading

BRANCH VEIN OCCLUSION STUDY GROUP (1984) Argon laser photocoagulation for macular oedema in branch vein occlusion. *American Journal of Ophthalmology*, **98**, 271–282

BRANCH VEIN OCCLUSION STUDY GROUP (1986) Argon laser scatter photocoagulation for prevention of neovascularisation and vitreous haemorrhage in branch vein occlusion. *Archives of Ophthalmology*, **104**, 34–41

BROWN, C. G. and MARGARGAL, L. E. (1979) Sudden occlusion of the retinal and choroidal circulations in a youth. *American Journal of Ophthalmology*, **88**, 690–693

CLEARY, P. E., WATSON, P. G., McGILL, J. and HAMILTON, A. M. (1978) Visual loss due to posterior segment disease in scleritis. *Transactions of the Ophthalmic Society of the UK*, **95**, 297–300

DODSON, P. M., GALTON, D. J., HAMILTON, A. M. and BLACH, R. K. (1982) Retinal vein occlusion and the prevalence of lipoprotein abnormalities. *British Journal of Ophthalmology*, **66**, 161–164

DODSON, P. M., WESTWICK, J., MARKS, G., KAKKAR, V. V. and GALTON, D. J. (1983) Thromboglobulin and platelet factor 4 levels in retinal vein occlusion. *British Journal of Ophthalmology*, **67**, 143–146

HAMILTON, A. M., KOHNER, E. M., ROSEN, D., BIRD, A. C. and DOLLERY, C. T. (1979) Experimental retinal branch vein occlusion in rhesus monkeys. I. Clinical appearances. *British Journal of Ophthalmology*, **63**, 377–387

HAYREH, S. S. (1971) Posterior ciliary arterial occlusive disorders. *Transactions of the Ophthalmological Society of the UK*, **91**, 291–303

HAYREH, S. S. and BAINES, J. A. B. (1972) Occlusion of the posterior ciliary artery I–III. *British Journal of Ophthalmology*, **56**, 719–764

HITCHINGS, R. A. and SPAETH, G. L. (1976) Chronic retinal vein occlusion in glaucoma. *British Journal of Ophthalmology*, **60**, 694–699

HOCKLEY, D. J., TRIPATHI, R. C. and ASHTON, N. (1979) Experimental retinal branch vein occlusion in rhesus monkeys. III. Histopathological and electron microscopical studies. *British Journal of Ophthalmology*, **63**, 393–411

LAATIKAINEN, L. and BLACH, R. K. (1977) Behaviour of the iris vasculature in central retinal vein occlusion: a fluorescein angiographic study of the vascular response of the retina and the iris. *British Journal of Ophthalmology*, **61**, 272–277

LAATIKAINEN, L., KOHNER, E. M., KHOURY, D. and BLACH, R. K. (1977) Panretinal photocoagulation in central retinal vein occlusion: a randomised controlled clinical study. *British Journal of Ophthalmology*, **61**, 741–753

MAY, D. R., KLEIN, M. L. and PEYMAN, G. A. (1976) A prospective study of xenon arc photocoagulation for central retinal vein occlusion. *British Journal of Ophthalmology*, **60**, 816–818

ORTH, D. and PATZ, A. (1978) Retinal branch vein occlusion. *Survey of Ophthalmology*, **22**, 357–376

ROSEN, D. A., MARSHALL, J., KOHNER, E. M., HAMILTON, A. M. and DOLLERY, C. T. (1979) Experimental retinal branch vein occlusion in rhesus monkeys. II. Retinal blood flow studies. *British Journal of Ophthalmology*, **63**, 388–392

RYAN, S. J. (1989) *Retina*, Vol. II, Chapters 73–75, C. V. Mosby, New York

SHILLING, J. S. and JONES, C. A. (1984) Retinal branch vein occlusion: A study of argon laser photocoagulation in the treatment of macular oedema. *British Journal of Ophthalmology*, **68**, 196–198

SHILLING, J. S. and KOHNER, E. M. (1976) New vessel formation in retinal branch vein occlusion. *British Journal of Ophthalmology*, **60**, 810–815

SPOLAONE, R., GAUDRIC, A., COSCAS, G. and deMARGERIE, J. (1984) Acute sectorial choroidal ischaemia. *American Journal of Ophthalmology*, **98**, 707–716

TROPE, G. E., LOWE, G. D. O., McARDLE, B. M., et al. (1983) Abnormal blood viscosity and haemostasis in longstanding retinal vein occlusion. *British Journal of Ophthalmology*, **67**, 137–142

WILLIAMS, B. I. and PEART, W. S. (1978) The effect of posture on intraocular pressure of patients with retinal vein occlusion. *British Journal of Ophthalmology*, **62**, 688–693

5
Small vessel and capillary disorders

Retinal capillary diseases

Diabetic retinopathy

Diabetic retinopathy has become one of the most common and time-consuming disorders faced by ophthalmologists. This is the result not only of an increase in the incidence of diabetes but also the fact that treatment has been shown to confer considerable benefit. Diabetic retinopathy is responsible for 8% of blindness registrations and is the commonest cause of blindness in those of working age in Western societies.

The incidence of diabetes is estimated to be between 1% and 2% of Western populations and has been shown to be on the increase in younger age groups. Diabetic retinopathy will probably be encountered more frequently in the future if current trends continue. There are many factors influencing the development of diabetes. The most common associations are a family history of diabetes, obesity, high alcohol consumption, and lack of exercise. Other associations include HLA type (B8, B15, Dw3, Dw4 in insulin dependency), certain racial groups (especially North American Indians), autoimmune endocrine disorders and possible virus infections (mumps, coxsackie B and rubella).

The diabetic population is broadly divisible into two groups: one third are type 1 (insulin dependent) and two thirds type 2 (non-insulin dependent). The majority of type 1 patients are younger (juvenile onset) whereas type 2 are older (maturity onset) but these age divisions are arbitrary; some patients developing diabetes later in life require insulin for diabetic control and some younger patients can be adequately controlled with oral hypoglycaemic agents. The prevalence of diabetic retinopathy in type 1 diabetics is twice that of type 2 (Table 5.1) but, once established, the clinical manifestations, progress and treatment are the same for both groups.

Table 5.1 Percentage of diabetic patients with retinopathy

Retinopathy	Diabetes	
	Type 1	Type 2
Background	31	16
Maculopathy	8	4
Proliferative	6	1
Advanced	2	0.2

Pathogenesis

Duration of diabetes has been conclusively shown to be a major influence on the development of retinopathy. For type 1 diabetics attending a diabetic clinic 20% of patients demonstrate retinopathy after 5 years of the disease, rising to 80% after 20 years. Similarly for type 2 diabetics 15% have retinopathy at 5 years and 50% at 15 years. Age of onset of diabetes in type 1 or type 2 is not significant for development of retinopathy.

The role of blood glucose control in the development of retinopathy has been disputed. The weight of evidence suggests that tight blood glucose control delays the onset of retinopathy but it is not known whether high average levels of blood glucose or fluctuations in levels are responsible for inducing the vascular changes.

Once retinopathy becomes established the influence of glucose control is not well understood. Hyperglycaemia induces high blood flow in the retinal circulation and lowering blood glucose from high levels decreases retinal blood flow. It has been shown that retinopathy of poorly controlled diabetics may become worse if blood glucose is suddenly reduced and kept within normal levels, for instance by a continuous subcutaneous infusion insulin pump. Short-term studies indicate treatment by insulin pump to control blood glucose rigidly leads to worsening of retinopathy although in the long term the severity of retinopathy may be lessened by tight control. Rapid reduction of blood flow may increase retinal capillary closure where vessel damage has occurred, but the subsequent more normal glycaemia prevents further capillary changes.

The biochemical defect inducing retinal capillary changes is not well understood. Increased aldose reductase activity producing high intracellular sorbitol levels has been suggested as a possible cause of pericyte loss.

Early histological changes show thickening of the retinal capillary basement membrane and reduction in the number of pericytes (mural cells) (Figure 5.1). Endothelial cells are initially spared but later proliferate causing microaneurysms. More extensive damage leads to capillary closure producing dilatation of adjacent collateral channels and development of intraretinal microvascular abnormalities. Aneurysmal dilatation and loss of the inner blood–retinal barrier between endothelial cells allows intravascular lipids and plasma to leak into the neuroretina causing chronic oedema and exudate formation. Capillary rupture produces small haemorrhages, mainly in the inner and outer plexiform layers of the neuroretina.

When capillary closure is extensive, retinal hypoxia leads to endothelial cell proliferation and penetration through the internal limiting lamina. This starts initially as solid buds but later canalization occurs forming capillary complexes. With further growth the capillaries lay down fibrous tissue around the vascular channels and develop into mature vessels. These fibrovascular changes are known as proliferative retinopathy and affected patients are at great risk of suffering serious loss of vision (see p. 34).

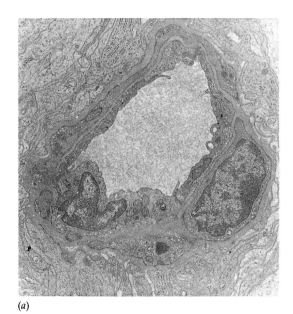

(a)

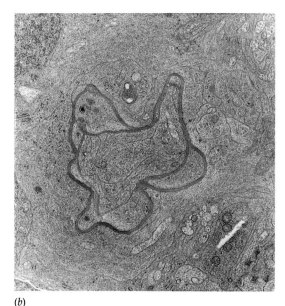

(b)

Figure 5.1 (a) Transmission electron micrograph of a normal retinal capillary. (b) Electron micrograph of a capillary affected by diabetic retinopathy. Note thickening of the basement membrane, loss of the pericytes and endothelial cell proliferation occluding the lumen compared with normal appearance. (Courtesy of Professor J. Marshall)

Clinical features

Background retinopathy The earliest changes observed ophthalmoscopically in the fundus are occasional microaneurysms and a few dot haemorrhages (minimal retinopathy). Such changes do not affect vision and are asymptomatic, but once retinopathy is present it is rare for patients to revert to normal.

Minimal retinopathy may remain static for many years or may progress to more severe background changes (Figure 5.2). Haemorrhages become more numerous and hard exudates are deposited. Unless a parafoveal capillary rupture causes a haemorrhage at the fovea, vision is not affected by background retinopathy and does not require treatment.

Diabetic maculopathy Patients become aware of gradual loss of central visual acuity. Usually this progresses over a period of months but sometimes deterioration of vision can occur over a few weeks. Three types of maculopathy can be identified: exudative, oedematous and ischaemic.

1. *Exudative maculopathy* causes progressive loss of central vision from deposition of lipid exudate around the fovea (Figure 5.3). Frequently such exudates develop in a circinate pattern from a central leaking area of abnormal capillaries and microaneurysms, but widespread capillary leakage may occur with multiple patches of exudate around the posterior pole of the retina. Exudates have a tendency to wax and wane but, if a persistent increase of lipid deposit is noted around the fovea, photocoagulation should be carried out, preferably before central visual loss occurs. Acuity, once lost, may not be regained after treatment.

2. *Oedematous maculopathy* causes gradual reduction of visual acuity from chronic foveal oedema. Loss of the inner blood–retinal barrier allows plasma fluid to accumulate in the neuroretina and, when the fovea is affected, vision progressively deteriorates. Exudates may also be present in these cases but not invariably so (Figure 5.4). In the majority of cases of oedematous maculopathy the leakage is focal and the points of capillary abnormality can be identified. In a few cases leakage can be from diffuse loss of the blood–retinal barrier over the whole capillary bed around the posterior pole but such cases are relatively rare. Macular oedema is most easily identified by contact lens examination at the slit lamp. Long-standing oedema is usually easily seen, with loss of retinal detail, thickening of the neuroretina and sometimes cystic foveal spaces. However, early or mild oedema can be difficult to recognize with only slight retinal thickening. Fluorescein angiography can sometimes be helpful in the diagnosis by demonstrating leakage around the fovea. Oedematous maculopathy should be treated by laser photocoagulation, preferably before acuity is seriously reduced.

3. *Ischaemic maculopathy* results in severe loss of central acuity from capillary closure around the macula. The vessels in the neuroretina become

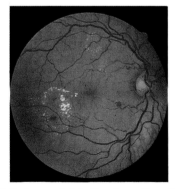

Figure 5.2 Background diabetic retinopathy with microaneurysms, punctate haemorrhages and lipid exudates

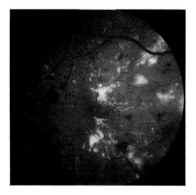

Figure 5.3 Diabetic maculopathy (exudative) with heavy lipid deposit around the fovea

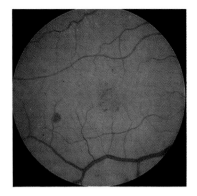

(a)

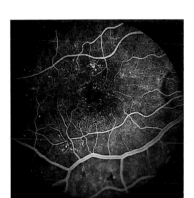

(b)

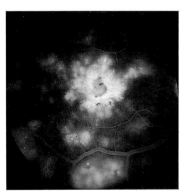

(c)

Figure 5.4 (*a*) Diabetic maculopathy (oedematous) showing foveal oedema. (*b*) and (*c*) Angiograms of (*a*) showing extensive capillary changes and fluorescein leakage at the macula

threadlike or absent and the retina becomes featureless and thinned from atrophy of the inner layers (Figure 5.5). Laser photocoagulation is not helpful in restoring visual acuity; however capillary closure at the macula is usually part of more extensive closure in the retinal periphery. These patients have a high risk of developing proliferative retinopathy at a later date and should, therefore, be closely watched for signs of new vessel formation.

Proliferative retinopathy   Closure of retinal capillaries induces hypoxia and release of neovascular factors. The capillary loss usually begins in the mid-periphery of the retina and then extends both anteriorly and posteriorly. New vessels proliferate in response to the neovascular factor and are

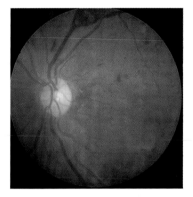

(a)

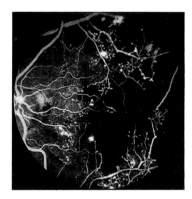

(b)

Figure 5.5 (*a*) Diabetic maculopathy (ischaemic). (*b*) Angiogram of (*a*) demonstrating extensive macular capillary closure

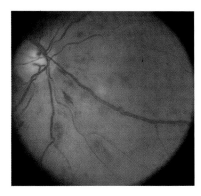

(a)

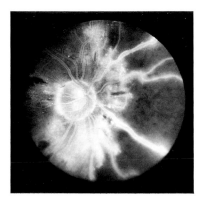

(b)

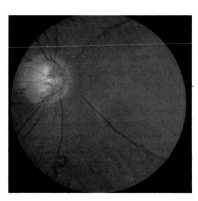

(c)

commonly found arising from the optic disc or from the upper and lower temporal venous arcades (Figures 5.6 and 5.7). They may, however, be found anywhere in the fundus and generally sprout from the border of perfused and non-perfused retina (Figure 5.8). The new vessels grow between the internal limiting lamina of the retina and the cortical gel of the vitreous. The vitreous subsequently detaches from the retina except in areas of increased adhesion and the new vessels remain and proliferate on the posterior surface of the vitreous (Figure 5.9).

Patients are usually unaware of visual symptoms in the presence of proliferative retinopathy until complications supervene. Traction from vitreous movement causes haemorrhage from the friable new capillary vessels and leads to sudden visual loss which may vary from a few floaters to complete, prolonged loss of all useful sight.

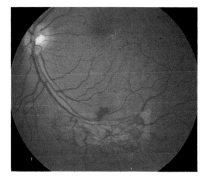

Figure 5.7 New vessels arising in peripheral retina

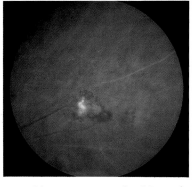

Figure 5.6 (a) Ischaemic diabetic retina nasal to optic disc: note vessel sheathing, venous beading and featureless retina. (b) Angiogram of (a) showing marked capillary closure. (c) Same view as (a) 6 months later, showing optic disc new vessels

Figure 5.8 Proliferative new vessels arising at the junction of perfused and non-perfused retina

Well-established neovascularization is accompanied by fibrosis around the endothelial channels which subsequently contracts and mature collagen is deposited. The contraction process causes traction on the retinal surface and on the posterior hyaloid face which remains adherent to areas of the retina, especially over the larger retinal vessels. Persistent traction causes retinal puckering, dragging of the macula and traction retinal detachment with accompanying loss of vision.

Proliferative retinopathy must always be looked for in longstanding diabetics because the threat to vision is serious and may be permanent. Photocoagulation is of proven benefit and must be given when active new vessel formation is present. When there are extensive signs of retinal ischaemia but there is no neovascularization, the retinopathy is often described as being in a preproliferative state. The presence of venous loops or beading, intraretinal diffuse haemorrhages, sheathing of arterioles or cotton wool spots indicate underlying retinal ischaemia, and careful observation is required in case neovascularization develops subsequently.

Advanced diabetic eye disease   The end-stages of ischaemia from diabetic retinopathy are known as advanced diabetic eye disease. These changes are present in approximately 1% of diabetics and follow untreated severe ischaemia or occur in eyes unresponsive to photocoagulation. Several manifestations can be identified:

1. Vitreous haemorrhage causes sudden disturbance in vision which, depending on the density of the haemorrhage, varies from mild floaters to complete loss of useful function (Figure 5.10).

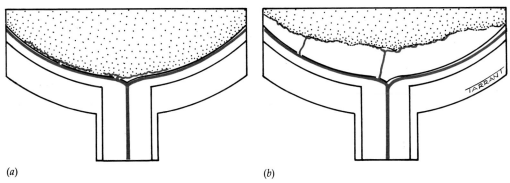

(a)   (b)

Figure 5.9 (a) Diagram of early proliferative new vessels arising at the optic disc and periphery growing between the retina and vitreous. (b) Vitreous detachment with new vessels adherent to and proliferating on the posterior hyaloid face

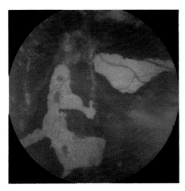

Figure 5.10 Severe retrohyaloid haemorrhage from optic disc neovascularization

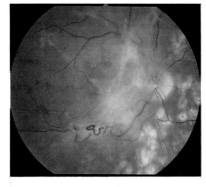

Figure 5.11 Diabetic fibrovascular tissue causing traction detachment and dragging of the macula

In most cases haemorrhage results from vitreous traction on active, fragile new vessels but may occur also from persistent vitreo-retinal traction in previously treated or quiescent proliferative retinopathy. Isolated vitreous haemorrhages often clear spontaneously during a period of months unless dense intragel blood is present. Untreated active neovascular tissue usually gives rise to recurrent vitreous haemorrhages.

2. Traction retinal detachment results from vitreo-retinal fibrous adhesions. Posterior vitreous separation leads to bridges of fibrovascular tissue across the post-hyaloid space with resulting bands stretching from the optic disc or peripheral retina to the posterior hyaloid face. Subsequent contraction of the fibrous tisssue causes the posterior hyaloid face to become taut from the vitreous base to the retinal adhesions and is followed by retinal distortion and detachment (Figure 5.11). Visual function is lost from distortion or detachment of the macula. Traction detachment may become rhegmatogenous if the fibrovascular adhesions cause a retinal tear.

3. Total retinal ischaemia is a rare form of advanced eye disease. The retinal vessels appear as thin white threads in an atrophic retina with absence of new vessels or traction detachment. Visual function is always very poor but treatment is useless (Figure 5.12).

4. Rubeosis iridis is induced by percolation of neovascular factors into the aqueous. Fibrovascular tissue is produced and extends over the surface of the iris, frequently occluding the drainage angle. Rubeotic glaucoma follows resulting in a red, irritable, painful eye (Figure 5.13).

Investigations

The majority of patients with diabetic retinopathy have been diabetic for many years, and the diagnosis is well established. Occasionally type 2 diabetics present with loss of vision as the first symptom and the clinical appearance of the retinopathy leads to the diagnosis. Urine testing for glucose and blood glucose estimation will confirm the diagnosis. Glycosylated haemoglobin or fructosamine levels may be useful in monitoring long-term glucose control if there is doubt about the adequacy of diabetic treatment.

Fluorescein angiography is not usually necessary in the management of most patients with retinopathy. The diagnosis is rarely in doubt and the progress of the retinopathy can be adequately followed by serial colour photography. In some cases of maculopathy angiography can be helpful in identifying ischaemia or areas of leakage which persist after laser treatment. Angiography or fluoroscopy can also help in confirming the presence of new vessels when there is doubt; the latter is particularly useful when moderate vitreous haemorrhage partially obscures the view of the fundus.

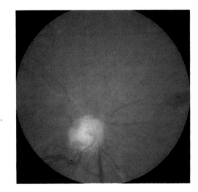

Figure 5.12 Gross retinal ischaemia from advanced diabetic retinopathy in the absence of proliferative retinopthy

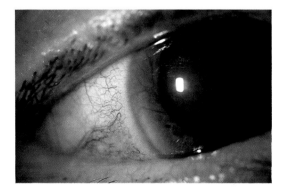

Figure 5.13 Rubeosis iridis and glaucoma secondary to diabetic retinopathy

Treatment

The mainstay of treatment of sight-threatening retinopathy is photocoagulation. Tighter control of blood glucose may delay the onset of retinopathy but only exceptionally leads to resolution of established changes.

Diabetic maculopathy   Photocoagulation reduces leakage into the retina from the defective inner blood–retinal barrier. Microaneurysms and haemorrhages from ruptured capillaries are treated directly with 100 μm laser spots with enough energy to produce a slight visible change in the vascular abnormality.

Exudates do not affect visual acuity until the central fovea is involved by deposit. Once exudates are observed to be increasing within approximately one third of a disc diameter of the fovea treatment should be carried out. Exudative maculopathy resolves in nearly all cases but recurs within 5 years in 35% of patients. Continued observation and treatment are, therefore, necessary. Visual acuity is usually maintained at the pretreatment level, hence the importance of early treatment before serious loss of acuity occurs. Occasionally a fovea affected with a heavy exudate deposit may improve considerably, with useful improvement of visual acuity (Figure 5.14), and treatment can be well worth undertaking in such cases.

Macular oedema responds to focal treatment similar to the technique used for exudative maculopathy, especially in younger patients (Figure 5.15). In 15% of elderly type 2 diabetics macular oedema persists in spite of resolution of the visible microvascular abnormalities. In such cases and in eyes with diffuse capillary leakage grid photocoagulation can be tried. Recurrence of oedema occurs in 9% of cases within 5 years and requires further treatment.

Proliferative retinopathy   Active neovascularization of the optic disc should be treated with

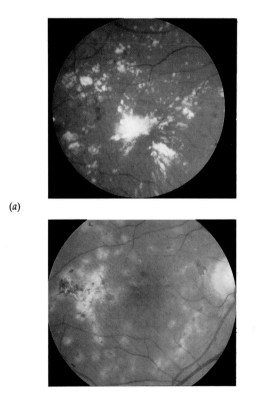

(a)

(b)

(c)

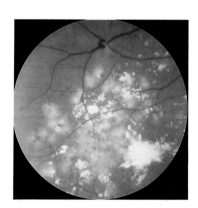

Figure 5.14 Exudative diabetic maculopathy – (*a*) pretreatment. (*b*) Immediately after laser treatment. (*c*) 15 months after laser treatment – note resolution of exudate

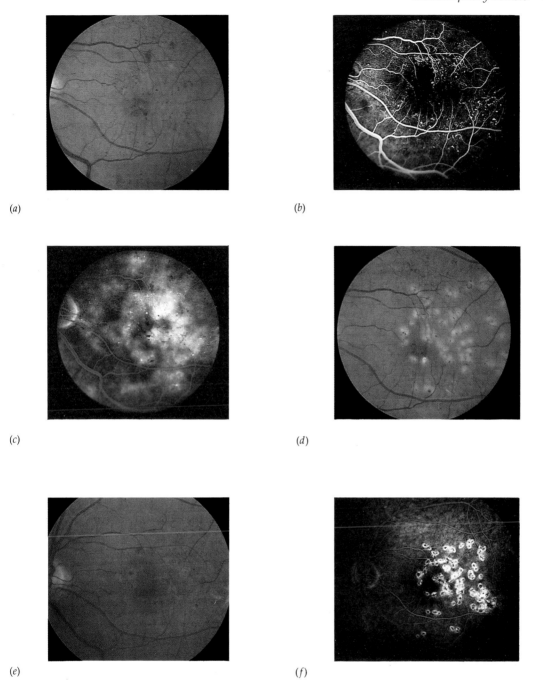

(a)

(b)

(c)

(d)

(e)

(f)

Figure 5.15 Oedematous diabetic maculopathy – (*a*) pretreatment. (*b*) and (*c*) Venous and late phase angiogram of (*a*). (*d*) Retinal appearance after laser treatment. (*e*) 1 year post treatment. (*f*) Late phase angiogram of (*e*) – note resolution of leakage

panretinal photocoagulation over the whole peripheral retina, sparing only the area around the macula, i.e. between the upper and lower temporal arcades and from the disc to the fovea and an equal distance temporal to the fovea (Figure 5.16). Treatment should be continued as anteriorly as possible with the three-mirror contact lens. The initial aim is to place approximately 2000–2500 laser applications of 500 μm over the fundus with 500 μm gaps between the burns; the precise number varies depending on the size of the eye and ease of application. When a panfundoscopic contact lens is used laser burns of 500 μm increase in size to 800 μm; therefore, fewer applications are necessary to produce the same effect. Some patients are able to tolerate the whole treatment in one session but if this is not possible the therapy can be given in two or three divided sessions. For those patients who experience great discomfort from laser treatment a retrobulbar injection of local anaesthetic can be helpful but topical anaesthesia

is usually sufficient for most patients. Retreatments tend to be more painful and retrobulbar anaesthetic is more frequently necessary.

Peripheral retinal new vessels do not carry quite the same severe risk of visual loss as disc new vessels but none the less often lead to vitreous haemorrhage and should be treated. An isolated focus of peripheral vessels can be treated by scatter photocoagulation in a sector of the retina peripheral to the neovascularization (Figure 5.16b). Multiple foci of peripheral vessels can be treated with a similar sectorial approach but it is usually better to administer panretinal photocoagulation similar to cases of disc new vessels. In time, many cases of peripheral vessels require multiple sectorial treatments and panretinal photocoagulation at the outset is more likely to prevent vitreous haemorrhage in the long term.

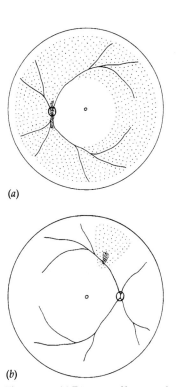

(a)

(b)

Figure 5.16 (*a*) Diagram of laser application for disc new vessels avoiding the macula and major vessels. (*b*) Sectorial laser treatment for peripheral new vessels

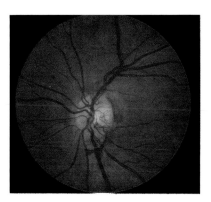

(a)

(b)

Figure 5.17 (*a*) Early proliferative disc new vessels. (*b*) After laser treatment – note complete regression of new vessels

After treatment a month should be allowed for the effect to become established. If new vessels remain active after this time resolution is not likely and a further laser session should be undertaken with another 1500 applications in those areas not previously covered.

Early new vessels usually regress and may disappear completely (Figure 5.17) but more established vessels become inactive and leave behind white fibrous tissue (Figure 5.18). Once neovascularization is inactive further photocoagulation is not necessary and is often contraindicated as contraction from residual fibrous tissue may increase and lead to traction retinal detachment. Once quiescent, proliferative retinopathy may remain inactive for prolonged periods but continued observation is necessary as long-term recurrences can occur.

Some cases of neovascularization continue to remain active in spite of repeated full courses of argon and xenon photocoagulation exceeding a total of 6000 or 7000 burns. The visual outlook for these very active cases is poor because even if the proliferative retinopathy is ultimately controlled progressive ischaemia of the retina leads to neuronal loss. Heavy treatment by laser photocoagulation reduces both colour perception and peripheral visual field, complications even more pronounced when xenon arc treatment is used.

A few diabetic patients develop retinopathy including proliferative changes in the far periphery of the retina near the equator. In such cases the areas of ischaemia are in the anterior retina with relative sparing posteriorly. Treatment

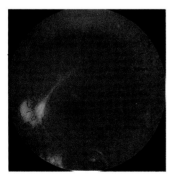

Figure 5.18 Residual fibrosis following vessel regression after laser treatment

of these extreme anterior areas can be difficult by laser and impossible by xenon. Under such circumstances peripheral cryotherapy can be used with good effect but caution must be exercised. Cryotherapy may lead to traction retinal detachment and is safer when used in divided sessions and repeated if necessary. Cryotherapy may also be used if vitreous haemorrhage has occurred from proliferative retinopathy and the view of the retina is obscured to such an extent that photocoagulation is not possible. The risk of retinal detachment is significant and it is usually better to wait for the haemorrhage to clear spontaneously and perform photocoagulation later. This may not be possible in cases of repeated haemorrhage and cryotherapy can be considered, particularly if rubeosis iridis is present. If the retina cannot be viewed directly, frequent ultrasound examinations are necessary to detect the presence of retinal detachment.

Advanced diabetic eye disease Persistent vitreous haemorrhage can be removed by vitrectomy but, unless both eyes are affected, several months should be allowed for spontaneous haemolysis. If active vessels are later revealed laser treatment should be given. When haemorrhage partly obscures the view of the fundus krypton laser photocoagulation, which is not absorbed by vitreous blood, can sometimes be effective where argon fails to produce sufficient reaction. In some cases vitreous haemorrhage recurs before an adequate view of the fundus is obtained and endolaser photocoagulation combined with vitrectomy offers the best chance of preserving useful vision. Vitreous haemorrhage may arise from persistent fibrous traction on the retina rather than from active neovascularization. Recurrent haemorrhages from continued traction require vitrectomy and release of the fibrous tissue.

Traction retinal detachment is a sinister complication of proliferative retinopathy. Provided no retinal breaks develop, traction detachments may remain static for months or years. If the detachment remains peripheral, visual function is not seriously impaired and surgery is not required. If the macula is affected by detachment or if a retinal tear develops, surgery becomes necessary and a vitrectomy combined with release of all retinal traction is needed. The techniques employed are beyond the scope of this book but cases of traction retinal detachment often require internal subretinal fluid drainage, internal tamponade and laser endophotocoagulation as well as vitrectomy and fibrous membrane excision (Figure 5.19).

Early rubeosis iridis should be treated in order to prevent the intractable painful glaucoma that may follow. Panretinal photocoagulation should be tried but peripheral cryotherapy can also be used. Once glaucoma is established portex tube drainage offers hope of preservation of useful vision but when function is very poor atropine and steroid drops are the treatment of choice. Enucleation may be necessary for a persistently painful eye.

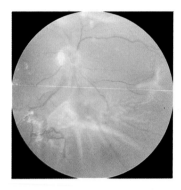

Figure 5.19 Traction retinal detachment following proliferative diabetic retinopathy

Systemic hypertensive retinopathy

Although hypertension is a systemic disorder mainly affecting larger blood vessels it has been included in this chapter because it is the retinal capillary changes that are important to the ophthalmologist.

Pathogenesis

Systemic hypertension has a variety of causes (e.g. renal disease, phaeochromocytoma, idiopathic) but the retinopathy resulting from raised blood pressure has the same features regardless of cause. Chronic, mild hypertension leads to compensatory thickening of the muscle and fibrous tissue layers of the arteriolar walls and damage to the microcirculation only occurs when the blood pressure becomes markedly elevated. More acute elevations of blood pressure as in malignant hypertension or acute renal disease produce capillary damage in the retina and optic nerve before compensatory arteriolar changes can develop.

Clinical features

Traditionally hypertensive retinopathy has been divided into four grades.

Grade I   – arteriolar tortuosity, thinning and silver wiring.
Grade II – Grade I plus arterio-venous nipping.
Grade III – Grade II plus haemorrhages, lipid exudates and cotton wool spots.
Grade IV – Grade III plus optic disc oedema

For ophthalmologists this classification is not helpful because it does not relate to any therapeutic approach to patients and confuses the underlying pathological process. It is better to consider hypertensive retinopathy as either compensated (benign) or decompensated (potentially visually threatening). The decompensated state may be either chronic focal leakage or acute focal hypoperfusion and infarction.

The *compensated retinopathy* encompases grades I and II of the traditional classification. There is arteriolar muscular hyertrophy leading to an increase in both width and length of the arterioles. Their appearance becomes tortuous with a heightened central reflex and, if the hypertrophy becomes severe, the visible blood column becomes thinner and irregular. Where arterioles cross venules the common adventitial sheath prevents the veins becoming displaced and the thickened arterial wall indents the venule. The veins become either nipped or cross arterioles at a more perpendicular angle (Figure 5.20). When protective arteriolar hypertrophy is insufficient the capillary bed develops focal areas of *decompensated retinopathy*. Initially this shows as areas of capillary leakage or closure resulting in scattered flame-shaped haemorrhages in the nerve fibre layer, lipid exudate deposition and patchy retinal oedema (Figure 5.21). Patients are not usually aware of visual disturbances unless the perifoveal capillaries are affected and the fovea develops chronic oedema or deposition of hard exudates. Such changes cause gradual deterioration of central visual acuity.

Acute decompensation of focal areas of the capillary bed from severe hypertension cause microinfarction with the appearance of cotton wool spots (Figure 5.21). Closure of the retinal capillaries produces axonal damage and rapid disturbance of the vision when the nerve fibres serving central vision are affected. Malignant hypertension induces fibrinoid necrosis of small arterioles and widespread ischaemia in both the retina and optic nerve. With optic nerve involvement patients become aware of fluctuating obscurations of vision which may then proceed to severe optic nerve infarction. The hallmark of malignant hypertension is optic disc oedema and patients demonstrating disc swelling should have urgent treatment not only to preserve vision but to prevent serious renal damage or cerebrovascular complications.

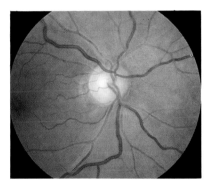

Figure 5.20 Compensated hypertensive retinopathy

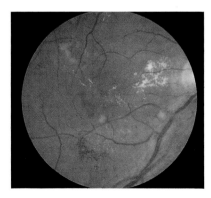

Figure 5.21 Decompensated hypertensive retinopathy – note lipid exudates, haemorrhages and microinfarcts

Investigations

The simple measurement of blood pressure is usually sufficient to establish the diagnosis in those patients with signs of retinal changes. When optic disc oedema is present the urine normally contains protein as a result of concurrent renal involvement and renal function must be assessed. Fluorescein angiography is not usually helpful in cases of hypertensive retinopathy but may be used to document areas of focal capillary disruption or confirm the presence of disc oedema if there is doubt.

Treatment

Compensated hypertensive retinopathy does not require treatment because vision is not threatened. If the blood pressure is considered to be significantly elevated referral to a physician will be necessary in case other systemic complications develop.

Decompensated retinopathy in which there is a threat to central vision from exudate, chronic oedema or infarction should be treated by lowering blood pressure. Cases showing cotton wool spots or optic disc oedema should always be referred for blood pressure control.

Once the systemic blood pressure is controlled the signs of exudate, oedema and cotton wool spots resolve and local treatment for the retina is not required. Vision usually recovers well unless macular oedema is longstanding or unless there is considerable neuronal loss at the fovea.

Associated conditions

Two retinal vascular conditions are recognized in patients with systemic hypertension:

1. Retinal branch vein occlusion. This is the commonest presentation of patients to ophthalmologists as a result of raised blood pressure. Venous embarrassment at arterio-venous crossings leads to impaired flow and occlusion (see p. 27). When branch vein occlusions occur in the presence of hypertension the blood pressure should be lowered to prevent further occlusive episodes in the same or fellow eye.
2. Retinal arteriolar macroaneurysms are associated with systemic hypertension (see p. 88).

Involutional sclerosis

Hypertensive retinopathy should be differentiated from involutional sclerosis resulting from ageing. In many elderly patients the ophthalmoscopic appearance of the retinal arterioles becomes thinned and sometimes irregular. This may resemble hypertensive arteriolar changes but the vessels are attenuated and there are no significant arterio-venous crossing changes. Occasional small retinal haemorrhages may occur but widespread exudation or ischaemia are absent. The arteriolar walls lose their muscle component and there is an increase in the fibrous tissue coat.

Venous stasis retinopathy

This relatively uncommon condition follows hypoperfusion of the retina secondary to reduction in blood flow in the internal carotid or ophthalmic artery. Atheromatous disease of the carotid artery is much the most common cause but other conditions such as pulseless disease can be seen rarely. The reduced ocular blood flow gives rise to a picture not dissimilar to central retinal vein occlusion but the severity of the signs depends on the degree of retinal ischaemia.

Clinical features

Mild cases of venous stasis show scattered dot retinal haemorrhages, particularly in the retinal periphery, and areas of capillary dilatation and tortuosity. Vision is often undisturbed initially but patients may become aware of a gradual loss of visual acuity.

More severe cases show signs of retinal ischaemia with a picture similar to central vein occlusion. The disc is often hyperaemic and swollen, haemorrhages become numerous and vascular sheathing and closure follow. Optic disc neovascularization is a frequent accompaniment in pronounced retinal ischaemia (Figure 5.22). When severe ocular ischaemia is present, as in ophthalmic artery occlusion, anterior segment complications may also develop. The eye becomes hypotonic with a heavy flare in a deep anterior chamber and may develop neovascular glaucoma.

Investigations

Light digital pressure on the eye produces collapse of the central retinal artery observable on ophthalmoscopy and is a helpful diagnostic sign. Ophthalmodynamometry will confirm the low arterial perfusion pressure.

Carotid ultrasonography is a useful non-invasive technique allowing carotid flow assessments in the neck. Arteriography can also be used to outline carotid and ophthalmic artery patency.

Treatment

Treatment of the primary cause of low perfusion should be considered if carotid artery obstruction is identified, and a specialist opinion sought. Carotid endarterectomy can restore perfusion in suitable cases but it is not possible to relieve ophthalmic artery obstruction. Peripheral vasodilator drugs have no proven benefit.

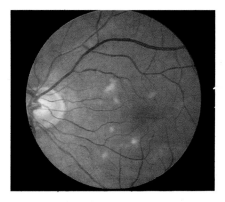

(a)

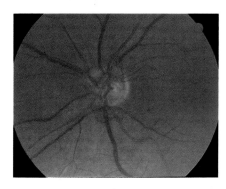

(b)

Figure 5.22 (*a*) Cotton wool spots secondary to carotid artery stenosis. (*b*) Disc neovascularization secondary to venous stasis retinopathy

Optic disc neovascularization, although carrying a much better prognosis than disc neovascularization in diabetes, should be treated by panretinal photocoagulation to prevent vitreous haemorrhage. It should be remembered that many of these patients have generalized vascular disease and are not suitable candidates for anaesthesia and vitrectomy. Therefore, it is important to regress neovascularization before vitreous haemorrhage occurs.

Carotid-cavernous fistula

Arterio-venous fistulae can occur either spontaneously or following head trauma. True carotid-cavernous fistulae are relatively uncommon and produce intense venous engorgement of the ipsilateral orbit and sometimes the contralateral orbit also. More commonly the fistula occurs between a dural artery and the cavernous sinus producing a less florid picture.

Increased pressure within the venous system leads to arterialization of the vein walls and may cause reduced perfusion within the eye. The patient presents with a clinical picture similar to venous stasis retinopathy and ocular ischaemia but the central retinal artery pressure remains normal. A bruit can sometimes be heard by the patient on auscultation of the head and dilated episcleral vessels are a pathognomonic sign (Figure 5.23).

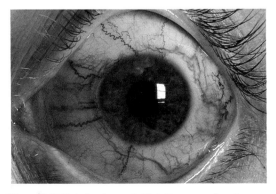

Figure 5.23 Episcleral vessel dilatation secondary to carotico-cavernous fistula

Peripheral occlusive disorders

There are a number of disorders which primarily affect the peripheral retinal circulation although in advanced cases the central retina can also be affected. The retina may be affected as a result of a systemic abnormality (e.g. S-C disease) but often no such disorder is apparent outside the eye (e.g. dominant exudative vitreo-retinopathy).

Sickle cell retinopathy

The globin fraction of haemoglobin has a characteristic sequence of amino acids which is directly inherited. Normal adult haemoglobin is designated haemoglobin A. Certain black races, particularly those from West Africa, the Caribbean and the United States of America have a high prevalence of abnormal genes concerned with haemoglobin production. Some individuals inherit a gene which substitutes a valine molecule in place of glutamic acid – i.e. the sickle or 'S' gene – in the beta globin fraction. When present the sickle gene leads to the carrier producing haemoglobin A-S (sickle trait) or if inherited from both parents, haemoglobin S-S (sickle cell disease). A similar abnormality also exists which substitutes lysine for glutamic acid causing another variation of the globin molecule – haemoglobin C. Combinations of these genes can occur producing haemoglobin S-C which is of particular interest to ophthalmologists as it produces retinal vascular abnormalities.

Haemoglobin S causes red blood cells to become inelastic and irregular when deoxygenated leading to capillary obstruction. S-S disease causes severe anaemia but has a low rate of retinopathy whereas S-C patients have less severe anaemia but a high incidence of retinal capillary obstruction. The rigid deformed red blood cells form rouleaux which impact in the retinal capillaries.

Clinical features The characteristic signs of sickle retinopathy occur near the equatorial retina with closure of the peripheral retinal vessels, arterio-venous anastamoses and foci of neovascularization – so-called sea-fans, which contain variable amounts of actively growing and fibrotic vessels. The new vessels are the result of peripheral retinal ischaemia and proliferate from the border of perfused and non-perfused retina (Figure 5.24). Although these new vessels are relatively slow growing, vitreous haemorrhages and traction retinal detachments may occur.

Stages of sickle retinopathy (Goldberg):

1. Peripheral vascular closure.
2. Peripheral circumferential arterio-venous anastamoses.
3. Peripheral new vessels.
4. Vitreous haemorrhage.
5. Traction retinal detachment.

Other features of retinal S-C disease include capillary abnormalities around the macula with an increase in the area of the capillary free zone, and patches of pigmentation in the retinal pigment epithelium known as sun-burst spots. Sun-burst spots have been considered to be a result of choroidal infarction but this is unlikely in view of the large diameter of the choroidal capillaries. Choroidal infarction has not been demonstrated histologically.

Treatment   The treatment of S-C retinopathy has been controversial. The relatively benign prognosis has been used as a reason for observing patients unless vitreous haemorrhage supervenes but in some patients bleeding becomes severe with complete loss of vision. Further treatment can become difficult without vitrectomy but, because general anaesthesia can produce systemic vascular occlusion, surgery should be avoided if possible in sickle cell patients. It is easier to treat patients with active neovascularization before they bleed, and extensive new vessels should have photocoagulation. Small areas can be watched and treated if they extend.

The basis of treatment, as with other forms of neovascularization, is to regress the active capillaries by reducing the effect of the neovascular factors from the hypoxic retina. Photocoagulation can be effective but treatment of the extreme retinal periphery can be difficult because of poor visualization of the anterior retina. In such cases peripheral cryotherapy to the retina or to the base of the sea-fans may be tried. This can usually be done with subconjunctival local anaesthetic and if extensive areas require treatment the therapy is best done in divided sessions.

Areas of old fibrosis do not need treatment as the risk of haemorrhage is relatively small and post-treatment contraction of the fibrous tissue may induce traction retinal detachment. It should also be borne in mind that retinal detachment surgery involving encircling procedures carries a

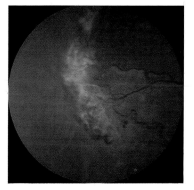

(*a*)

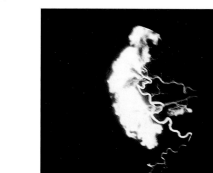

(*b*)

Figure 5.25 (*a*) Peripheral retinal neovascularization in S-Thal disease. (*b*) Angiogram of (*a*) showing closure peripheral to the new vessels which leak profusely

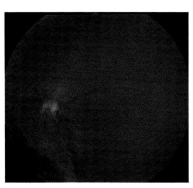

Figure 5.24 Peripheral retinal neovascularization in S-C disease

significant risk of anterior segment ischaemia and subsequent necrosis.

Thalassaemia is another inherited haemoglobulinopathy which affects the production of the globin fraction of haemoglobin. In itself thalassaemia does not affect the retinal circulation but when combined with sickle trait (S-thal), a retinopathy similar to S-C disease results (Figure 5.25).

Retinopathy of prematurity (retrolental fibroplasia)

Premature babies requiring post-natal support in an incubator are at risk of developing a characteristic retinopathy affecting the peripheral retina. Babies at particular risk are those of very low birth weight (less than 1500 g), extreme prematurity and those given high oxygen concentrations to overcome their respiratory distress.

In the years following the identification of retinopathy of prematurity (ROP) the incidence steadily declined but the introduction of better neonatal care has allowed more premature babies of lower birth weight to survive. As a result the number of potential cases of ROP has risen over the past few years.

The peripheral retina of the fetus is not vascularized until just before full term. In the premature infant the peripheral retina is, therefore, avascular and post-natal high oxygen concentration induces closure of the developing terminal retinal vessels. The vessel tips become necrotic, and following restoration of normal oxygen concentrations vascularization of the immature retina does not proceed. The mechanism whereby oxygen causes vessel closure is not fully understood but may be either a direct toxic effect on immature retinal vessels or from increased choroidal oxygen reducing the requirement for retinal vascularization.

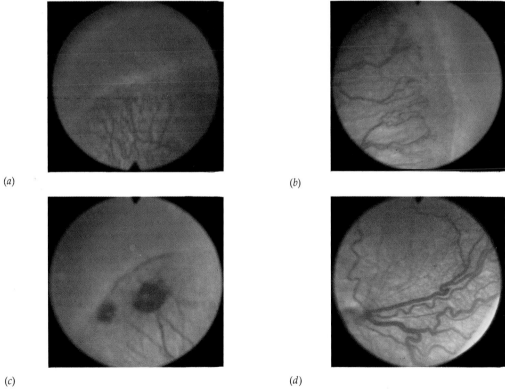

(a)

(b)

(c)

(d)

Figure 5.26 Retinopathy of prematurity. (*a*) Stage 1. (*b*) Stage 2 with fibrous ridge. (*c*) Stage 3 with new vessels. (*d*) ROP 'plus' with posterior vessel tortuosity. (Reproduced by courtesy of Mr E. Schulenburg.)

Clinical features ROP has an acute phase followed by a cicatricial stage. It should be remembered that in a normal infant the peripheral retina does not become vascularized until 8–9 months of gestation and when examining the peripheral fundus blood vessels will not be seen in a premature baby.

ROP develops at around 32–36 weeks gestational age, with abnormal peripheral retinal arborizations and a line of demarcation at the limit of vascularization. Haziness in the peripheral vitreous is also seen. The acute phase may resolve completely or progress through a number of recognizable stages and can result in bilateral blindness.

Stages of ROP (Figure 5.26).

1. Demarcation line between vascularized and non-vascularized retina with abnormal peripheral terminal vessels.
2. Stage one with the addition of a fibrovascular ridge of intraretinal tissue at the demarcation line.
3. Stage two plus fibrovascular proliferation into the cortical vitreous from the ridge.
4. Stage three plus localized traction retinal detachment originating from the area of the fibrous ridge.
5. Total retinal detachment

Different areas of the fundus may show different stages of the disease and the number of clock hours involved is important when assessing prognosis. The posterior retina may also show an increased vascular tortuosity (ROP 'plus') and when present carries a worse outlook for vision (Figure 5.26).

Myopia, which may be severe, is a constant feature of ROP. Because the fibrotic reaction is more pronounced in the temporal periphery the neuroretina is pulled temporally producing an ectopic macula and characteristic dragging of the nasal vessels around the temporal edge of the optic disc. Although ROP is mainly a vascular disorder, loss of retinal ganglion cells has also been reported following high oxygen concentrations in premature infants.

Occasionally mild forms of ROP may present several decades later with vitreous haemorrhages or rhegmatogenous retinal detachment. Posterior vitreous detachment in the myopic eyes of ROP patients causes traction on the residual fibrovascular tufts in the equatorial retina which then bleed or form retinal tears. Dragging of the optic disc or peripheral retinal signs in the fellow eye usually provide the key to the diagnosis.

Treatment The large majority of babies with ROP do not require treatment. When needed, treatment is by cryotherapy to the peripheral avascular retina and the area of the ridge and new vessels. If acute ROP appears progressive during the weeks after birth with the development of stage 3 disease cryotherapy should be applied. Acute ROP often regresses and stages 1 and 2 should be observed carefully as the signs may not progress, but active preretinal new vessels should be treated. Retinal detachment requires scleral buckling but if fibrosis is marked a vitrectomy may also be needed. Severe traction detachments have been approached by open sky and closed vitrectomy but the visual results are not good.

The role of vitamin E supplements as an anti-oxidant in the prevention of ROP in at-risk babies has not been well defined to date.

Dominant exudative vitreo-retinopathy

This rare condition resembles retinopathy of prematurity in the appearance of the peripheral fundus. However, unlike ROP there is no relevant history of prematurity, postnatal care in an incubator nor oxygen administration. The disorder is inherited in an autosomal dominant pattern and the patients are not usually myopic.

Clinical features.

Different family members demonstrate a wide variation in the severity of retinopathy. Mild cases show peripheral vascular closure with straightening of the surviving retinal vessels immediately posterior to the avascular region. Intermediate cases have equatorial fibrovascular proliferation but severe involvement induces marked peripheral fibrous traction with retinal detachment. The vessels at the disc appear dragged and the visual acuity is reduced depending on the degree of macular ectopia. The condition is bilateral.

Eales disease and retinal vasculitis

Eales disease, as originally described, consists of recurrent vitreous haemorrhages in young men. It is now established that the cause of the recurrent haemorrhages is neovascularization secondary to peripheral retinal capillary closure and it is not confined exclusively to males. The underlying aetiology of the vascular closure is unknown but a similar clinical picture has been observed in certain cases of retinal vasculitis of known aetiology (see Chapter 8). The term Eales disease is probably best restricted to those cases in whom the aetiology is unknown and where there is no active inflammation. Although this distinction between Eales disease and retinal vasculitis may be artificial in some cases, it simplifies the therapeutic approach because anti-inflammatory drugs do not influence Eales disease but may be important in active retinal vasculitis.

An association between tuberculosis and Eales disease has long been described, particularly in the Indian subcontinent. Whether this is a true association or just a result of chance in an area of high prevalence is not proven but tuberculosis can cause retinal vasculitis. Once the inflammatory process resolves the peripheral retinal vessels remain occluded and secondary neovascularization may occur. Such cases should be categorized as tuberculous vasculitis rather than Eales disease and, as the understanding of the mechanisms of this and similar conditions expands, the number of cases of unknown aetiology labelled 'Eales disease' will gradually diminish.

Clinical features

Some patients are asymptomatic but others are aware of floaters in their vision for months or even years until the onset of vitreous haemorrhage.

A detailed description of the retinal vascular changes in cases of vasculitis are outlined in Chapter 8, but in Eales disease the peripheral retina is avascular with sheathed or ophthalmoscopically absent arterioles and venules. New vessels originate either from the surviving peripheral circulation or sometimes from the optic disc (Figure 5.27a).

Investigations

These should be undertaken to exclude known causes of retinal vasculitis, particularly tuberculosis, sarcoidosis, Behçet's disease and the collagenoses. If positive, appropriate medical treatment should be instigated (see Chapter 8).

Treatment

Neovascularization in the absence of active vasculitis should be treated with retinal photocoagulation or cryotherapy. Initially this should be concentrated in the retinal periphery but sometimes it is necessary to carry out full panretinal photocoagulation (Figure 5.27b).

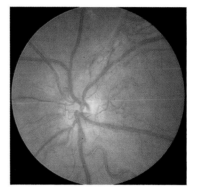

(a)

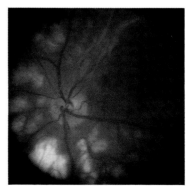

(b)

Figure 5.27 (a) Eales disease and disc new vessels. (b) 1 year after panretinal photocoagulation

Vitreous haemorrhage should be allowed to clear spontaneously for several months unless both eyes have lost vision. Vitrectomy may be necessary but there is a risk of retinal detachment from peripheral fibrovascular traction on areas of thin, atrophic retina.

Choroidal capillary diseases

Systemic hypertension and eclampsia

Severe elevations of systemic blood pressure as in malignant hypertension or eclampsia may produce closure of branches of the short ciliary arteries within the choroid. This appears to be a separate entity from hypertensive retinopathy and may occur in the absence of retinal vascular changes.

Clinical features

Widespread multifocal choroidal vessel occlusions produce scattered infarcts of the retinal pigment epithelium. Patchy whitish-grey lesions are visible with overlying secondary serous retinal datachment: vision is correspondingly severely reduced (Figure 5.28). A similar clinical picture has been described in association with thrombocytopenic purpura and intravascular coagulopathy.

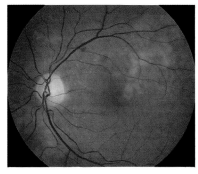

Figure 5.28 Acute choroidal infarction in severe hypertension: note RPE pallor in upper temporal quadrant

Fluorescein angiography

This confirms the multifocal nature of the choroidal pigment epithelial disturbance. There is patchy non-perfusion of the choroid and areas of slow filling. Late staining of the pigment epithelium follows with subsequent diffuse dye leakage into the subretinal space.

Treatment

Control of blood pressure leads to spontaneous resolution of the secondary retinal detachment. The appearance of the retinal pigment epithelium returns to normal or remains with patchy pigmentary changes. Vision usually returns to near normal but severe choroidal infarction may limit recovery.

Retinal pigment epitheliopathies

This group of disorders is suspected rather than known to be of vascular origin and includes acute posterior multifocal placoid pigment epitheliopathy, Harada's disease and geographic chorioretinopathy.

Acute posterior multifocal placoid pigment epitheliopathy (APMPPE)

This relatively uncommon disorder usually affects young adults of either sex. Sometimes there is a history of mild systemic infection or antibiotic administration 2 or 3 weeks previously but many cases occur without obvious cause. It has been suggested that an immune mechanism is involved but this is not proven and immune complexes have not been identified. Normally the condition is bilateral but unilateral cases are described.

Clinical features Discrete grey–white plaque-like lesions are visible at the level of the retinal pigment epithelium. The plaques are usually ⅛–¼ of a disc diameter (Figure 5.29). In some cases there are a few white cells visible in the vitreous and in severe cases shallow secondary detachment of the overlying neuroretina can be seen. Vision is mildly reduced unless the fovea is directly affected by a plaque.

Fluorescein angiography Angiography shows early hypofluorescence over the white plaques in the pigment epithelium. This may represent infarction and failure of individual choriocapillaris lobules to fill or possible masking of the underlying choroid by the thickened pigment epithelial cells. Late in the fluorescein run the plaques stain mildly and the optic disc is sometimes hyperfluorescent (Figure 5.29).

Systemic investigation is unrewarding but evidence of recent infection or immune abnormalities can be looked for.

Treatment The condition is self-limiting and visual recovery is normally complete but sometimes a subfoveal plaque will permanently reduce visual acuity. The pigment epithelium returns to near normal ophthalmoscopically but shows focal disturbance on angiography.

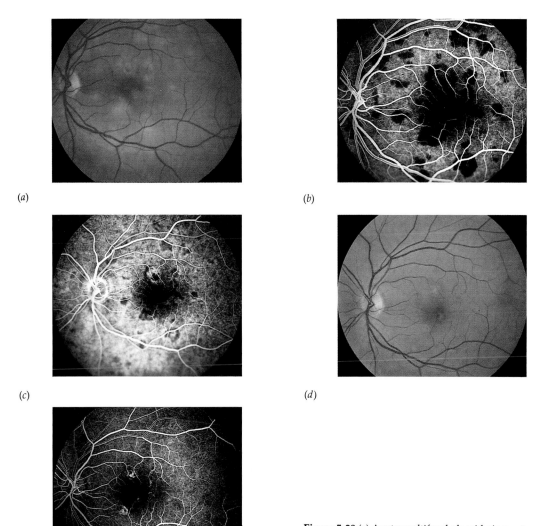

(a)

(b)

(c)

(d)

(e)

Figure 5.29 (*a*) Acute multifocal placoid pigment epitheliopathy. (*b*) and (*c*) Angiograms of (*a*) showing delayed filling of choroidal lobules underlying pale patches of RPE. (*d*) Resolution of (*a*) showing slight pigment epithelial disturbance. (*e*) Angiogram of (*d*) with normal choroidal filling and mild transmission defects

Harada's disease

Harada's disease is comprised of bilateral serous retinal detachment and signs of inflammation of the meninges or central nervous system. Some patients may also have vitiligo, poliosis and severe granulomatous anterior uveitis (Vogt–Koyanagi syndrome). The condition is more common in oriental and black races and may affect either sex. In view of the pigmentary changes of the VK-H syndrome and the histological similarity to sympathetic ophthalmia the aetiology is presumed to be an immunological reaction to melanin.

Clinical features   Harada's disease usually affects the posterior segment of the eye in the absence of other skin and anterior segment features. Typically the vitreous shows considerable cellular infiltration and the retinal pigment epithelium has large grey elevated patches (Figure 5.30). Extensive secondary exudative detachment of the neuroretina occurs with profound visual loss. The retina may become totally detached in severe cases.

Distinction between acute multifocal posterior placoid pigment epitheliopathy and Harada's disease can sometimes be difficult as the signs of the two disorders are similar. A severe case of AMPPE could be confused with a mild case of Harada's disease and it has been suggested that they form different ends of a spectrum of disease, possibly manifesting different racial susceptibilities.

Harada's disease must be differentiated from posterior scleritis which may have a similar fundus appearance but is often associated with pain and mild proptosis.

Fluorescein angiography   This has a characteristic appearance of irregular filling of the choriocapillaris and hypofluorescence over the areas of pigment epithelial elevation. As the dye transit progresses there is increasing hyperfluorescence under the pigment epithelium giving the typical lobular pattern (Figure 5.30) and also staining of the optic disc.

Patients with central nervous system signs should have a lumbar puncture to show the leucocytosis and high CSF protein. This is important if there is doubt concerning the diagnosis and if meningeal tumours such as reticulum cell sarcoma are suspected.

Treatment   In Caucasian patients the disease tends to run a relatively benign course but oriental races often have permanent severe loss of vision. Systemic steroids in high doses greatly increase the speed of resolution and are indicated in all but the mildest of cases.

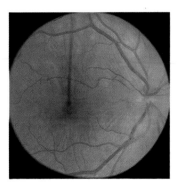

(*a*)

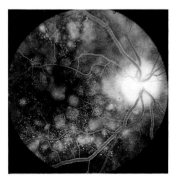

(*b*)

Figure 5.30 (*a*) Harada's disease – note secondary retinal detachment and retinal striae. (*b*) Angiogram of (*a*)

Serpiginous (geographic) chorioretinopathy

Geographic choroidopathy or chorioretinopathy must not be confused with geographic atrophy of the retinal pigment epithelium. The former is a relapsing pigment epitheliopathy and the latter an age-related atrophy (see Chapter 6).

Clinical features   Geographic choroidopathy can affect either sex and the patient is usually of middle age. Both eyes are normally involved but one eye can be considerably more affected than the other. No systemic association has been identified and the disease is worldwide.

Acute lesions often arise adjacent to old pre-existing burnt out areas of earlier attacks. The pigment epithelium shows one or more white patches approximately the size of the optic disc, sometimes with mild vitreous cellular infiltration and infrequently with overlying serous retinal detachment (Figure 5.31).

Initially the disease starts around the optic disc or posterior pole and over a period of months spreads peripherally as more acute lesions arise. Ultimately, the whole posterior fundus is severely affected by gross atrophy. Vision is affected in proportion to the degree of pigment epithelial loss; visual acuity is maintained until the fovea is affected by an acute lesion following which the central vision is lost. Retinal function in the affected areas is destroyed and the visual prog-nosis is poor. Secondary neovascular macular disciform lesions are common.

Fluorescein angiography Fluorescein angiography has a characteristic appearance. In common with the other retinal pigment epitheliopathies the acute lesions mask the underlying choriocapillaris, then stain with fluorescein as the transit progresses. Old lesions show well-demarcated patches of RPE atrophy with loss of the choroidal capillaries in the bed of the lesions; the larger choroidal vessels survive. The lesions appear relatively dark centrally with hyperfluorescent edges (Figure 5.31).

Treatment No treatment has been proven to be of benefit. If the fovea is threatened by an acute lesion systemic steroids can be tried but are usually ineffective.

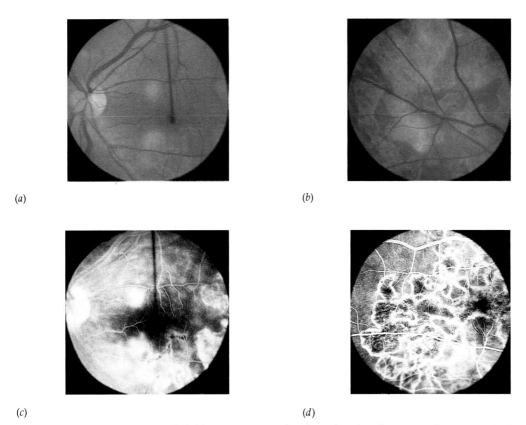

(a)   *(b)*

(c)   *(d)*

Figure 5.31 (*a*) Acute pigment epithelial lesions in geographic choroidopathy. (*b*) Longstanding geographic lesions in fellow eye of (*a*). (*c*) and (*d*) Angiograms of acute and chronic lesions of same patient

Further reading

AABERG, T. M. (1979) Clinical results in vitrectomy for diabetic traction retinal detachment. *American Journal of Ophthalmology*, **88**, 246–253

BRITISH MULTICENTRE PHOTOCOAGULATION TRAIL (1977) Proliferative diabetic retinoplasty: treatment with zenon arc photocoagulation. *British Medical Journal*, **i**, 739–741

CHISHOLM, I. H., GASS, J. D. M. and HUTTON, W. L. (1976) The late stage of serpiginous (geographic) choroditis. *American Journal of Ophthalmology*, **82**, 343–351

COGAN, D. G. (1975) Ocular involvement in disseminated intravascular coagulopathy. *Archives of Ophthalmology*, **93**, 1–8

COMMITTEE FOR THE CLASSIFICATION OF RETINOPATHY OF PREMATURITY (1984) An international classification of retinopathy of prematurity. *Archives of Ophthalmology*, **102**, 1130–1134

CRYOTHERAPY FOR RETINOPATHY OF PREMATURITY COOPERATIVE GROUP (1988) Multicentre trial of cryotherapy for retinopathy of prematurity. *Archives of Ophthalmology*, **106**, 471–479

DIABETIC RETINOPATHY STUDY RESEARCH GROUP (1978) Photocoagulation treatment of proliferative diabetic retinopathy. *Transactions of the American Academy of Ophthalmology and Otology*, **85**, 82–106

DUANE, T. D. *Clinical Ophthalmology*, Vol. III, Chapters 13, 16 and 17, Harper and Row, New York

FASTENBERG, D. M., FETKENHOUR, C. L., CHOROMOKOS, E. and SHOCH, D. E. (1980) Choroidal vascular changes in toxaemia of pregnancy. *American Journal of Ophthalmology*, **89**, 362–368

GAUDRIC, A., COCAS, G. and BIRD, A. C. (1982) Choroidal ischaemia. *American Journal of Ophthalmology*, **94**, 489–498

GOLDBAUM, M. H., FLETCHER, R. C. JAMPOL, L. M. and GOLDBERG, M. F. (1979) Cryotherapy of proliferative sickle retinopathy. *British Journal of Ophthalmology*, **63**, 97–101

GOLDBERG, M. F. (1971) Natural history of untreated proliferative sickle retinopathy. *Archives of Ophthalmology*, **85**, 428–437

GOLDBERG, M. F. and ACACIO, I. (1973) Argon laser photocoagulation of proliferative sickle retinopathy. *Archives of Ophthalmology*, **90**, 35–44

GREY, R. H. B. (1986) The treatment of diabetic maculopathy by argon laser photocoagulation. *Transactions of the Ophthalmological Society of the UK*, **104**, 424–430

GREY, R. H. B., MALCOLM, N., O'REILLY, D. and MORRIS, A. (1986) Ophthalmic survey of a diabetic clinic. I. Ocular findings. *British Journal of Ophthalmology*, **70**, 797–803

HAMILTON, A. M. (1978) Diabetic blindness and its prevention by photocoagulation. *Transactions of the Ophthalmological Society of the UK*, **98**, 296–298

HANSCOM, T. A. (1982) Indirect treatment of peripheral retinal neovascularisation. *American Journal of Ophthalmology*, **93**, 88–91

HERCULES, B. L., GAYED, I. I., LUCAS, J. B. and JEACOCK, J. (1977) Peripheral retinal ablation in the treatment of proliferative diabetic retinoplasty: a 3 year intensive report of a randomised, controlled study using argon laser. *British Journal of Ophthalmology*, **6**, 555–563

KEARNS, T. P. (1979) Ophthalmology and the carotid artery. *American Journal of Ophthalmology*, **88**, 714–722

KEEN, M., and JARRETT, J. (1982) *Complications of Diabetes*, Arnold, London

KINYOUN, J. L. and KALINA, R. E. (1986) Visual loss from choroidal ischaemia. *American Journal of Ophthalmology*, **101**, 650–656

KISSUN, R. D., HILL, C. R., GARNER, A., PHILLIPS, KUMAR, S. and WEISS, J. B. (1982) A low-molecular-weight angiogenic factor in cat retina. *British Journal of Ophthalmology*, **66**, 165–169

MICHELS, R. G. (1978) Vitrectomy for complications of diabetic retinopathy. *Archives of Ophthalmology*, **96**, 237–246

OBER, R. R., BIRD, A. C., HAMILTON, A. M. and SEHMI, K. (1980) Autosomal dominant exudative vitreo retinopathy. *British Journal of Ophthalmology*, **64**, 112–120

PALMBERG, P., SMITH, M., WALTMAN, S., *et al.* (1981) The natural history of retinopathy in insulin dependent juvenile onset diabetes. *Ophthalmology*, **88**, 613–618

PLUMB, A. P., SWAN, A. V., CHIGNELL, A. H. and SHILLING, J. S. (1982) A comparative trial of xenon arc and argon laser photocoagulation in the treatment of proliferative diabetic retinopathy. *British Journal of Ophthalmology*, **66**, 213–218

REESER, F., FLEISCHMAN, J., WILLIAMS, G. A. and GOLDMAN, A. (1981) Efficacy of argon laser photocoagulation in the treatment of circinate diabetic retinopathy. *American Journal of Ophthalmology*, **92**, 762–767

RICE, T. A., MICHELS, R. G. and RICE, E. F. (1983) Vitrectomy for diabetic traction retinal detachment involving the macula. *American Journal of Ophthalmology*, **95**, 22–33

RYAN, S. J. (1989) *Retina*, Vol. II, Chapters 103, 104, 106, C. V. Mosby, New York

SCHULENBURG, W. E., HAMILTON, A. M. and BLACH, R. K. (1979) A comparative study of argon laser and krypton laser in the treatment of optic disc neovascularization. *British Journal of Ophthalmology*, **63**, 412–417

SCHULENBURG, W. E., PRENDIVILLE, A. and OHRI, R. (1987) Natural history of retinopathy of prematurity. *British Journal of Ophthalmology*, **71**, 837–843

SCOBIE, I. N., MacCUISH, A. C., BARRIE, T., GREEN, F. D. and FOULDS, W. S. (1981) Serious retinopathy in a diabetic clinic: prevalence and therapeutic implications. *Lancet*, **ii**, 520–521

TAYLOR, C. M., WEISS, J. B., KISSUN, R. D. and GARNER, A. (1986) Effect of oxygen tension on the quantities of procollagenase-activating angiogenic factor present in the developing kitten retina. *British Journal of Ophthalmology*, **70**, 162–165

TOWNSEND, C., BAILEY, J. and KOHNER, E. (1980) Xenon arc photocoagulation for the treatment of diabetic maculopathy. *British Journal of Ophthalmology*, **64**, 385–391

WEST, K. M. (1978) *Epidemiology of Diabetes and Its Vascular Lesions*, Elsevier, Holland

WHITELOCKE, R. A. F., KEARNS, M., BLACH, R. and HAMILTON, A. M. (1979) The diabetic maculopathies. *Transactions of the Ophthalmological Society of the UK*, **99**, 314–320

YOUNG, N. J. A., BIRD, A. C. and SEHMI, K. (1980) Pigment epithelial diseases with abnormal choroidal perfusion. *American Journal of Ophthalmology*, **90**, 607–618

6

The ageing macula and disciform degeneration

Age-related macular degeneration is of great socio-economic importance in Western countries because it is the largest single cause of registrable blindness. Although relatively infrequent before the age of 65 thereafter it becomes very common and accounts for 30–50% of blind registrations affecting up to 120 per 100 000 of the population over the age of 70. The incidence also seems to be increasing even allowing for the demographic increase in the elderly population.

In common with all tissues of the body the retina undergoes degenerative and atrophic changes as a result of ageing. The neuroretinal layers become thinned, particularly in the periphery, and microcystic spaces often develop, which can subsequently coalesce to form senile schisis. The arrangement of the cell bodies of the neural layers of the retina may also become deranged with migration of nuclei into the plexiform layers.

The major ageing changes, however, are seen in the retinal pigment epithelium. This highly phagocytic tissue is required throughout life to digest vast quantities of discarded membrane discs from the outer segments of the retinal photoreceptors. The digested photoreceptor debris is transferred to the choriocapillaris through Bruch's membrane. With age the efficiency of the process becomes reduced, causing undigested material to accumulate within the pigment epithelial cells and Bruch's membrane. As a consequence of the ageing process the macula is subject to a variety of degenerative disorders with different histological and clinical manifestations.

Ageing macular atrophy

Pathogenesis

Ageing of the retina has been demonstrated to produce a sequence of histological changes, mainly affecting the photoreceptors, pigment epithelium and choriocapillaris. Bruch's membrane is particularly affected and becomes progressively disordered throughout life. In the young adult Bruch's membrane has an orderly arrangement consisting of five layers: basement membrane of the pigment epithelial cells, inner collagenous layer, elastic layer, outer collagenous layer and basement membrane of the endothelium of the choriocapillaris (Figure 6.1). As a result of

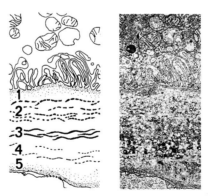

Figure 6.1 Bruch's membrane in young adult. 1 = RPE basement membrane; 2 = inner collagen layer; 3 = elastin layer; 4 = outer collagen layer; 5 = choriocapillaris basement membrane. (Reproduced by courtesy of Professor J. Marshall)

ageing the layers become disordered. Lipid material is deposited and large collagen bundles are laid down leading to overall thickening of Bruch's membrane, which may also contain macrophages (Figure 6.2). A layer of amorphous material can sometimes be observed at the level of the pigment epithelial basement membrane and is known as the basal linear deposit.

Accumulations of partially digested photoreceptor outer segment debris initially arise within the pigment epithelial cells but later become deposited between the pigment epithelial cells and Bruch's membrane forming microdrusen (Figure 6.2), which subsequently increase in size and become visible ophthalmoscopically. Histologically drusen form two different types: discrete drusen composed of hyalinized lipid material, often containing calcium, and diffuse drusen which are granular and contain protein and lipofuscin.

Drusen usually have a symmetrical distribution in both eyes. They tend to be clustered around the macula but sometimes they may be more widespread and not infrequently involve the retinal periphery (Figure 6.3). On occasions drusen are observed in the fundus close to the major retinal vessels with relative sparing of the macular area.

A third type of very fine drusen known as cuticular drusen has also been described (Figure 6.4). These are different from the drusen associated with ageing and are often inherited as an autosomal dominant disorder. They are probably thickenings of the pigment epithelial cell basement membrane and are much more easily seen on angiography than clinically (Figure 6.4). Although cuticular drusen do not affect vision patients are subject to the later formation of ageing drusen and associated macular disturbances and neovascularization.

With increasing failure of the metabolic processes involved in the catabolism of the photoreceptor discs, the pigment epithelial cells show lipofuscin deposition within the cell cytoplasm. Disorganization of the melanin granules and pigment clumping occurs and the cells undergo atrophy. The precise enzyme failure responsible for this degeneration has not been established.

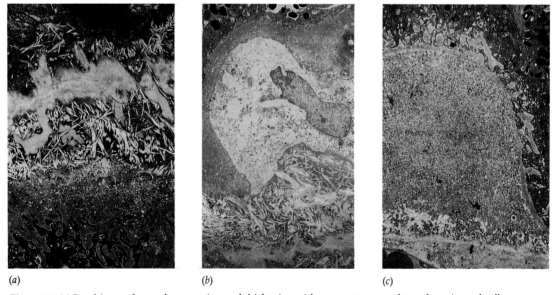

(a)   *(b)*   *(c)*

Figure 6.2 (*a*) Bruch's membrane degeneration and thickening with age – note amorphous deposits and collagen deposition. (*b*) Macrophage in Bruch's membrane. (*c*) Drusen material lying between RPE basement membrane and collagen layer of Bruch's membrane. (Reproduced by courtesy of Professor J. Marshall)

The changes in Bruch's membrane may render it impervious to the transport of pigment epithelial cell breakdown products to the choriocapillaris. Alternatively biochemical changes in the nature of the photoreceptor discs may render them indigestible to pigment epithelial cell breakdown or there could be failure in the enzymatic processes of the pigment epithelial cells themselves. Once the epithelial cells degenerate there is secondary atrophy of the photoreceptors.

The choriocapillaris may also be seen to be atrophic in those areas where the pigment epithelium is lost, especially when there is extensive degeneration present (geographic atrophy).

Clinical features

Some degree of atrophy of the macula is visible ophthalmoscopically in the eyes of most people over the age of 70. Often this amounts to no more than a few asymptomatic drusen. More extensive changes generate an increase in the number of drusen and there is clumping of melanin in the pigment epithelium. The drusen may be of the white, discrete crystalline variety (hard) or may be greyer and more diffuse (soft). When pigment epithelial cells undergo atrophy, pale patches become visible at the macula, but in spite of quite extensive changes visual acuity is often remarkably good (Figure 6.5).

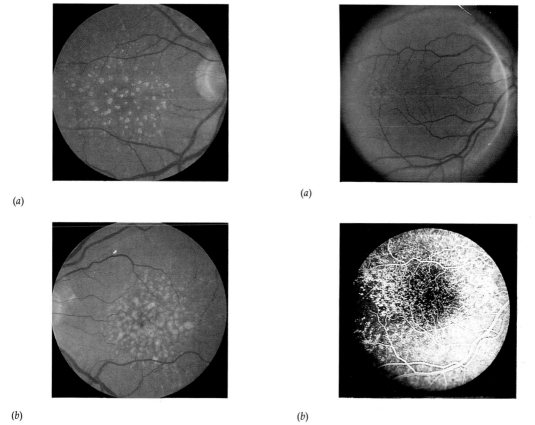

(a)

(b)

Figure 6.3 (*a*) Crystalline (hard) drusen. (*b*) Diffuse (soft) drusen

(a)

(b)

Figure 6.4 (*a*) Cuticular drusen. (*b*) Angiogram of (*a*) – note widespread disease not always well seen ophthalmoscopically

With increasing degeneration more extensive areas of the pigment epithelium become lost and secondary degeneration of the overlying photoreceptors causes gradual diminution of central vision. Eventually widespread areas of full-thickness atrophy of photoreceptors, pigment epithelium and choriocapillaris occur giving an appearance of sharply demarcated degeneration around the posterior pole of the eye and revealing the larger choroidal vessels in the bed of the lesion. This was formerly known as choroidal sclerosis but no true sclerosis of the choroidal vessels occurs and the condition is now known as geographic atrophy of the macula. In such cases central acuity is permanently and severely affected (Figure 6.6).

Fluorescein angiography is not usually required for patients with macular atrophy unless an associated neovascular disciform lesion is also suspected. The atrophic areas of the pigment epithelium show a transmission defect with hyperfluorescence of the underlying choriocapillaris (Figure 6.6). The hyperfluorescence fades as

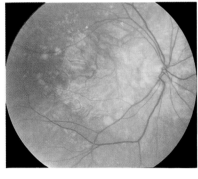

(a)

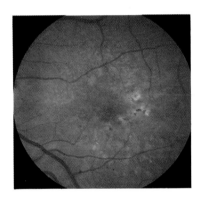

(a)

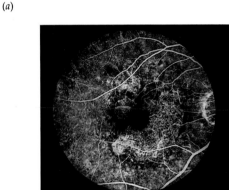

(b)

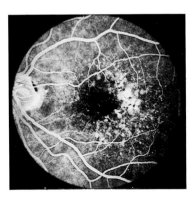

(b)

Figure 6.5 (a) Early atrophy of pigment epithelium with pigment clumping and drusen. (b) Angiogram of (a) showing transmission defect with no true leakage

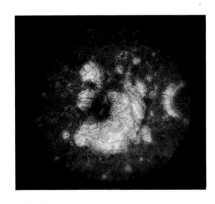

(c)

Figure 6.6 (a) Geographic atrophy of pigment epithelium. (b) Angiogram of (a) – note choriocapillaris filling. (c) Late phase angiogram of (a) showing transmission defect

the dye transit progresses and the fluorescein passes out of the ocular circulation. With extensive atrophy scleral staining is visible over areas of choriocapillaris loss.

Treatment

Because the basic defect in this condition is one of atrophy no active treatment is available which restores the continuity of the pigment epithelium to an intact, functional monolayer. Pigment epithelial cells are capable of replication *in vitro* but this does not occur following atrophy from ageing. Whether this is a result of metabolic changes from alterations in Bruch's membrane or because of atrophy of the choriocapillaris is unknown.

Elderly patients in whom visual acuity has been lost in both eyes often benefit from low vision aids and advice about lighting conditions. This can help them to utilize their residual vision for reading. Reassurance that only central vision will be affected is important and there is a large range of domestic aids available which can be invaluable in the home.

Vascular disciform degeneration

Age related

As a response to the ageing process some eyes develop choroidal neovascularization at the macula. This is a quite different response from the atrophic process described above although ageing changes in the pigment epithelium and in Bruch's membrane are the underlying cause. Unlike dry atrophic degeneration, subretinal or subpigment epithelial fluid develops at the macula and gives rise to a number of different clinical manifestations. The circular or oval serous elevation of the neuroretina is shown as disciform degeneration.

Pathogenesis

During the development of the neovascular process vessels grow from the choriocapillaris through Bruch's membrane. They proliferate either between Bruch's membrane and the pigment epithelium or penetrate the pigment epithelium and lie under the neuroretina destroying the outer blood retinal barrier (Figure 6.7). For this development it is necessary to have both a surviving choriocapillaris and disruption of Bruch's membrane. Eyes with multiple confluent soft drusen are at greater risk of developing a disciform lesion than those with hard discrete drusen. In the ageing eye it has been shown that there are multiple penetrations of Bruch's membrane by new vessels over widespread areas of the fundus including the periphery. Normally such vesssels do not proliferate but at the macula they may be triggered into active proliferation although the nature of the mechanism is unknown. Suggested factors include increase in the basal linear deposit, the presence of macrophages within Bruch's membrane, ischaemia of the outer

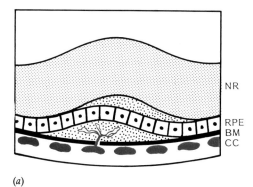
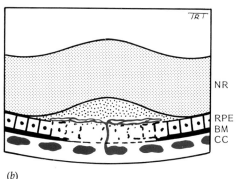

(a)   (b)

Figure 6.7 (*a*) Diagram of neovascular tissue penetrating Bruch's membrane and lying in the sub-pigment epithelial space. Fluid in subretinal space may also be present. NR = neuroretina; RPE = pigment epithelium; BM = Bruch's membrane; CC = choriocapillaris. (*b*) Neovascular tissue penetrating Bruch's membrane and pigment epithelium with overlying serous neuroretinal detachment

neuroretina, imperviousness of Bruch's membrane to a diffusable metabolite, altered immunity such as to retinal S antigen and accumulation of a vasogenic substance within Bruch's membrane. Pigment epithelial cells are capable of generating factors able both to induce and inhibit new vessel growth. Peripheral lesions sometimes occur but are rare, and the disciform response is almost exclusively a macular phenomenon.

Histologically new vessels have been shown to cross Bruch's membrane and affect the overlying pigment epithelium. As the vessels grow, a fibrotic reaction follows with destruction of the pigment epithelial cell layer and fluid accumulation under the neuroretina. Ultimately the lesion matures leaving a fibrovascular plaque of scar tissue which may involve a considerable area of the posterior pole of the eye (Figure 6.8).

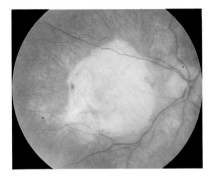

Figure 6.8 Large fibrotic disciform macular lesion

Clinical features

The development of a disciform lesion causes disturbance of central vision. Initially patients are aware of distortion of lines of print, kinking of straight edges and mild blurring of vision. After some weeks the acuity becomes further reduced

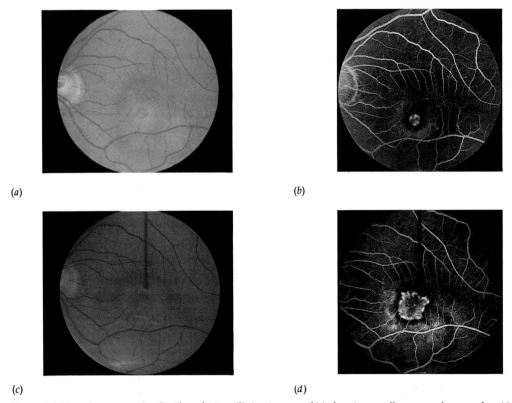

(*a*)

(*b*)

(*c*)

(*d*)

Figure 6.9 (*a*) Early neovascular disciform lesion. (*b*) Angiogram of (*a*) showing small neovascular complex. (*c*) Same eye 3 months later. (*d*) Angiogram showing growth of new vessels from foveal edge of original lesion to affect fovea

and patients frequently complain of a blank patch in the middle of the vision of the affected eye. An Amsler chart often allows patients to demonstrate the size and position of the retinal disturbance.

Examination of the fundus in the presence of an early disciform lesion usually reveals a circular or oval area of subretinal fluid involving the fovea and a smaller pink or greyish patch at the level of the pigment epithelium (Figure 6.9). The characteristics of the fundus lesion depend on the behaviour of the neovascular complex and the time the process has been present.

Serial observations of a disciform lesion show that neovascularization usually originates eccentric to but within one and a half disc diameters from the fovea. After a few weeks the neovascular membrane expands outwards from the point of origin, particularly from the edge closest to the fovea. Sooner or later the foveal pigment epithelium becomes affected with considerable loss of central vision (Figure 6.9). The new vessels are friable and liable to rupture producing subretinal haemorrhage (Figure 6.10). When the vessels have been present for some time subretinal exudates may form under the retina (Figure 6.11) and variable quantities of fibrous tissue laid down. Disciform degeneration can, therefore, demonstrate a pleomorphic picture but the diagnosis is not usually difficult. The presence of subretinal fluid is a strongly suggestive sign and some form of ageing change is nearly always present in the fellow eye.

Ultimately the disease becomes inactive and involutes to leave a fibrous scar. The subretinal fluid absorbs but this may take a number of years. Following flattening of the neuroretina visual distortion often improves; visual acuity rarely recovers to any great degree although patients can sometimes see 6/60 using eccentric vision.

Fluorescein angiography

This can be extremely helpful in the diagnosis and management of disciform degeneration. Identification of the position and size of the neovascular complex is made much easier and in instances where photocoagulation is contemplated angiography is necessary in almost all cases.

The neovascular complex arises from the choriocapillaris and, therefore, fills with dye at the same time as the choroid, i.e. usually before the retinal capillary circulation. As the transit progresses the fluorscein escapes through the capillary walls causing increasing hyperfluorescence with intense leakage in the late stage of the angiogram (Figure 6.12). Subsequently, dye seeps into the subretinal space giving a diffuse hyperfluorescence over the area of the posterior pole elevated by subretinal fluid.

Some cases of disciform degeneration demonstrate multiple foci of dye leakage rather than a single neovascular membrane. Such cases represent numerous small neovascular invasions through Bruch's membrane and often affect wide areas of the posterior pole including the fovea (Figure 6.13).

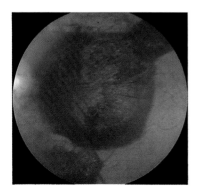

Figure 6.10 Haemorrhagic disciform lesion

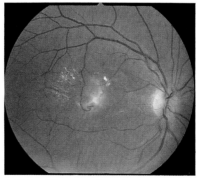

Figure 6.11 Small longstanding disciform lesion. Note subretinal exudate and also cilioretinal anastomosis

Treatment

A number of treatments have been proposed for ageing macular disease but with the exception of photocoagulation in selected disciform lesions none has been shown to be of material benefit. Lipid mobilizing agents such as clofibrate enjoyed popularity for a while and oral steroids have been tried but there is no rationale for such approaches and they do not improve vision.

Laser photocoagulation has been shown to be helpful in selected instances. The rationale is based on eradication of the neovascular tissue and allowing the subretinal fluid to absorb. The treatment has to be carried out before the fovea becomes involved in the disease process and before central acuity is significantly damaged.

Studies have shown that the majority of early neovascular capillary complexes are eccentric to the fovea, theoretically allowing laser treatment without damaging the fovea. If patients are identified in the first 2 weeks of the disease, approximately 75% of lesions are treatable, whereas only 50% can be treated after a month and less than 30% by 3 months. After a year the likelihood of treatment being possible is less than 1% and at this late stage 75% of affected eyes have an acuity of 6/60 or less.

Patients identified with a disciform lesion should be considered for fluorescein angiography to assess the position and extent of the neovascular membrane. When visual acuity is poor or the lesion longstanding it is unlikely that treatment will be appropriate and further action is not

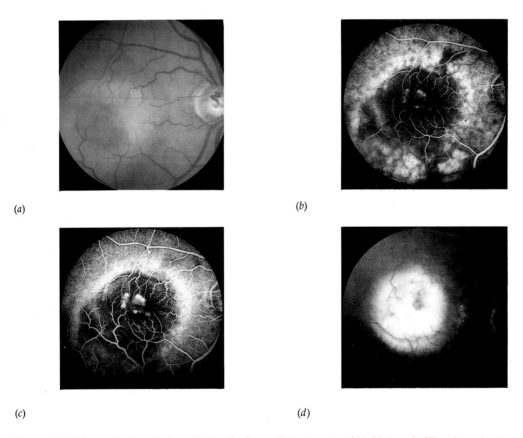

(a)

(b)

(c)

(d)

Figure 6.12 (a) Large disciform lesion affecting the fovea. (b) Angiogram of (a). Note early filling from choriocapillaris. (c) Increasing diffuse hyperfluorescence from new vessels. (d) marked leakage of fluorescein into subretinal space

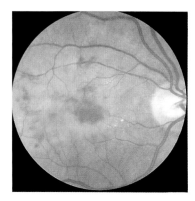

(a)

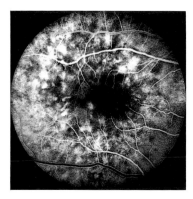

(b)

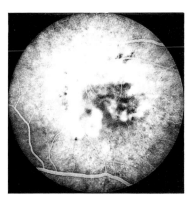

(c)

Figure 6.13 (*a*) Extensive disciform macular lesion. (*b*) and (*c*) Angiogram of (*a*) showing multiple foci of new vessel growth through Bruch's membrane

usually required. When visual acuity is good, particularly if 6/12 or better, or if the lesion has been present for a few weeks angiography should be carried out to assess the vascular details at the macula. Provided the new vessels can be identified and there is a definable space between the edge of the membrane and the foveola of 150 μm or more, laser photocoagulation can be considered. However, only in about half the cases will treatment be ultimately successful in obliterating the new vessel membrane. Patients should be aware of this prior to photocoagulation and also that the laser produces a dense scotoma which can be troublesome because of the proximity of the fovea.

Laser treatment is carried out with the intention of applying heavy, confluent photocoagulation burns over the whole neovascular lesion, overlapping the edges by 50 μm or so. If successful the new vessels will regress within a week or two and the subretinal fluid will absorb allowing preservation of central vision and abolition of annoying metamorphopsia. Visual acuity remains at the pretreatment level but further loss of central vision is prevented.

More recently it has been suggested that laser treatment may not obliterate the new vessels directly but allows the pigment epithelium to proliferate as an intact monolayer over the new vessels, confining them to the subpigment epithelial space. If this is ultimately shown to be the mechanism whereby treatment works then it may be better to cover the neovascular membrane by less heavy photocoagulation burns to allow more pigment epithelial cells to survive and replicate. This, however, is a theoretical approach based on experimental findings and is currently of unproven clinical benefit.

The most important single factor in preventing treatment of disciform degeneration is delay in referral and assessment of affected patients. Management should be based on early referral and angiography. This can be difficult to achieve in a hard pressed clinical service and with patients who are often uncomplaining and frequently do not realize the significance of their initially relatively mild symptoms. Ideally only a few days should pass from initial symptoms to having the processed angiogram to hand in order to see whether treatment is feasible. If a lesion is untreatable patients should be warned about the fellow eye which has a strong tendency to become similarly affected. Some 12–15% of fellow eyes are affected per annum (i.e. about 50% in 5 years) and patients should be instructed to seek help immediately if they become aware of visual disturbance in their second eye.

Once treatment is decided upon it should be carried out without delay. Topical anaesthesia is normally all that is required although some patients require a retrobulbar anaesthetic in order to prevent eye movement during treatment. The exact position of the fovea should be identified as far as possible and the area of the fundus requiring treatment must be found precisely by reference to the pattern of retinal vessels in the eye and on the angiogram. Once the area to be treated has been identified a single trial application of laser should be given to assess the response. This is best done with a 200 μm spot for 0.1 s on the edge of the membrane farthest from the fovea. The response of the patient to the laser and the reaction of the pigment epithelium can be assessed. The power setting on the laser can be adjusted to give a white burn by further trial shots and if the patient is intolerant of the treatment a retrobulbar injection can be used. The lesion is then covered by 200 μm burns for 0.2–0.5 s which should overlap each other and the edge of the new vessel membrane (Figure 6.14). A dense white burn is produced which then resolves into a full thickness pigment epithelial defect (Figure 6.14).

Because the treatment is carried out close to the fovea there is a tendency for the blue light of the laser to be absorbed by the luteal pigment, causing neuronal damage in the neuroretina. This can be greatly reduced by the use of green, yellow or red wavelengths either by the use of a filter in an argon laser or by using purpose-built dye or krypton lasers. It should be remembered that on a few occasions neovascular membranes bleed during treatment and that red wavelengths cannot be used to staunch further haemorrhage. Repeated firing of argon laser light at a small bleeding point will often prevent further haemorrhage.

Following treatment the outcome should be assessed after 2 weeks. Angiography at this time can be helpful but is not always necessary when the subretinal fluid has absorbed. If subretinal fluid persists or there is any question of continued activity of the treated lesion angiography must be repeated. Active new vessels should be retreated without delay according to the same principles involved in treating the original lesion and reviewed after a further 2 weeks. In the absence of activity another review at 1 month is advisable as the early recurrence rate is significant. Further activity or persistent subretinal fluid requires reassessment and the treatment pursued in the same way until either the new vessel membrane regresses or until it grows under the fovea and the lesion becomes untreatable. New vessels underlying the papillomacular bundle can be treated without fear of damaging the ganglion cell layer. The major area of energy uptake is in the pigment epithelium and choroid which is separated from the neuroretina by the layer of subretinal fluid.

After treatment has been successful and the lesion has resolved for 6–8 weeks the patient should be discharged with instructions to present immediately if there is a recurrence of symptoms. Follow-up appointments should not be given routinely as patients often wait for their allotted visit and, if there has been a recurrence, this causes delay and progression of the disease to an untreatable state. The rate of recurrence after treatment is similar for involvement of the second eye, namely 12–15% per annum, and patients must be warned that recurrences are common. Treatment only regresses the neovascular lesion and does not alter the underlying ageing disorder.

Patients who suffer bilateral severe visual loss due to subfoveal disciform lesions should be offered support services such as low vision aids, domestic appliances, talking books, mobility training where appropriate and the other social services available to the blind or partially sighted.

Disciform degeneration secondary to other disorders

Age-related pigment epithelial degeneration is by far the most common cause of choroidal neovascularization and is responsible for some 85% of all disciform lesions. However, it is now realized that almost any disease giving rise to damage or breaks in the retinal pigment epithelium and Bruch's membrane close to the fovea can subsequently allow development of the disciform process. In common with age-related lesions, neovascularization occurring around the macula has a similar tendency to grow towards the fovea, causing loss of central vision. The most common associations of secondary disciform lesions are myopia, pre-sumed ocular histoplasmosis syndrome, choroidal ruptures and diseases affecting the optic disc and surrounding pigment epithelium. Choroidal neo-vascularizaton has also been described in associ-ation with many other fundus diseases (Table 6.1).

Many of these associations are rare but several are encountered sufficiently commonly to merit special consideration. As in cases of ageing disciform degeneration the presenting symptom is usually blurred or distorted vision, and severe visual loss can occur when the subfoveal pigment

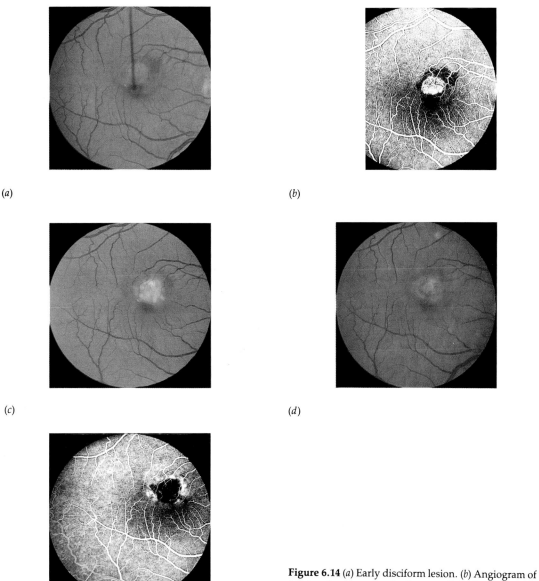

(a)

(b)

(c)

(d)

(e)

Figure 6.14 (*a*) Early disciform lesion. (*b*) Angiogram of (*a*) showing new vessels above capillary free zone. (*c*) Treatment photograph with overlapping laser applications. (*d*) and (*e*) 6 weeks after treatment with pigment epithelial defect and abolition of new vessels

Table 6.1 Macular disorders associated with secondary disciform lesions

Inherited disorders:
  Myopia
  Best's disease
  Pseudoxanthoma elasticum
  Cone dystrophy
  Rod–cone dystrophy
  Retinitis pigmentosa
  Polymorphic dystrophy
  Pseudo-inflammatory dystrophy of Sorsby
  Angioid streaks (sickle cell disease)
  Dominant drusen

Acquired pigment epithelial disorders:
  Choroidal rupture
  Presumed ocular histoplasmosis syndrome
  Geographic choroidopathy
  Acute multifocal placoid pigment epitheliopathy
  Harada's disease
  Toxoplasmosis
  Toxocariasis
  Parafoveal photocoagulation scars
  Rubella retinopathy
  Idiopathic neovascularization

Miscellaneous conditions:
  Choroidal osteoma
  Retinal venous occlusion
  Diabetic retinopathy
  Juvenile haemorrhagic maculopathy
  Choroidal naevus
  Birdshot choroidopathy

Optic disc disorders:
  Papilloedema
  Drusen
  Idiopathic peripapillary lesions

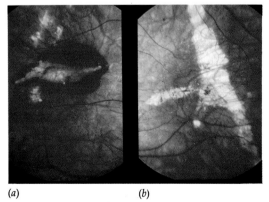

(a)   *(b)*

Figure 6.15 (*a*) Lacquer crack at the macula in high myopia. (*b*) Macular haemorrhage in high myopia unassociated with neovascularization

epithelium is disrupted. Patients with secondary lesions tend to be younger and the final visual prognosis is often better than in older patients. After the new vessels have reached the involutionary stage and the subretinal fluid has absorbed it can be expected that 60–70% of affected eyes will see 6/60 or better. The comparable figure for ageing disciform degeneration is only 30%.

Myopia

The macula in pathological myopia can be affected either by full-thickness atrophy of the retinal pigment epithelium, by subretinal haemorrhages from capillary rupture or by choroidal neovascularization. During the period of progression of high myopia the posterior pole becomes enlarged and in severe cases develops a staphyloma. The process of ectasia causes the inner layers to become stretched and thinned giving rise to the typical appearances around the optic disc of the crescent or annulus of absent Bruch's membrane and pigment epithelium. The choroid becomes attenuated and in time the macula also develops atrophic changes which may increase long after the myopia has stopped progressing. Myopia accounts for some 5–10% of blind registrations as a result of extensive chorioretinal atrophy of the macula but blindness is not common before the seventh or eighth decades of life.

Clinical features   Early atrophic changes are seen as linear breaks in the pigment epithelium (lacquer cracks) which slowly increase over a period of years into more widespread atrophy (Figure 6.15). Sometimes simple subretinal haemorrhages arise in the subretinal space causing disturbance of central vision which later absorb and vision returns to near normal (Figure 6.15). Haemorrhages can also develop at the macula as a result of underlying choroidal neovascularizaton and in such cases it is unusual for visual acuity to return to normal. Not all neovascular complexes bleed and many are visible as small greyish rings with overlying subretinal fluid at or close to the fovea known as the Foester–Fuchs' spot. In most instances Foester–Fuchs' spots arise under the fovea and remain small and circumscribed unlike the disciform lesions affecting the elderly. On occasions the new vessels arise eccentric to the fovea and may then expand to involve the fovea with corresponding reduction of visual acuity (Figure 6.16).

Treatment Lacquer cracks and simple macular haemorrhages require no treatment. Subfoveal Foester–Fuchs' spots should not be treated by laser photocoagulation because visual acuity will be further reduced by the post-treatment scotoma.

No statistical evidence exists which proves that eccentric disciform lesions in myopia should be lasered but clinical experience shows the new vessels often respond well to photocoagulation and thereby the threat to the fovea from expansion of the complex is reduced. Recurrences sometimes occur after treatment but are less common than in cases of ageing degeneration. Successful treatment produces morphological improvement and stabil-

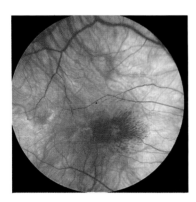

(a)

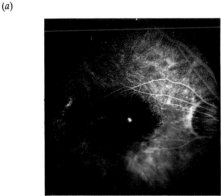

(b)

Figure 6.16 (*a*) Haemorrhage from Foester–Fuchs spot – note central new vessel complex. (*b*) Angiogram of (*a*) showing subfoveal new vessels

ity of vision in the majority of patients after abolition of the new vessels and absorption of the subretinal fluid.

Presumed ocular histoplasmosis syndrome (POHS)

This condition was first recognized in the United States of America, particularly around the Mississippi valley. The high prevalence of the fungus *Histoplasma capsulatum* and the fact that affected patients frequently had positive skin tests to Histoplasma antigens gave the syndrome its name. It is now recognized that the same clinical picture is found world wide and in areas where Histoplasma is not endemic, but the name persists.

Clinical features Patients of either sex may be affected and usually present in the fourth and fifth decades of life. A triad of ocular signs can be observed:

1. Peripapillary atrophy of the pigment epithelium.
2. Small, white discrete areas of pigment epithelial and choroidal atrophy in the peripheral fundus.
3. Disciform macular lesions (Figure 6.17).

Often pale pigment epithelial spots are found around the posterior pole and sometimes the peripheral lesions may be linear or confluent rather than punched out.

It is presumed that previous systemic infection by Histoplasma or some other organism causes subclinical spread to the choroid and leads to granulomatous lesions. These resolve but at a later date choroidal neovascularization occurs through an area of damaged Bruch's membrane near the fovea. In about 10% of patients the fundus develops further atrophic areas in the pigment epithelium in succeeding years and in approximately a quarter of cases the second eye also becomes affected.

Treatment Although the patients are younger than those affected by ageing disciform degeneration and therefore the prognosis for retention of useful vision is better, it has been shown that photocoagulation is beneficial in some cases. When the new vessels are close but do not affect the fovea photocoagulation to obliterate the neovascular complex increases the chances of retaining good central vision. Patients with subfoveal new vessels or simple atrophic areas should not be treated. Patients with new vessels more than a disc diameter from the fovea can be watched initially in case there is no extension of the capillary network towards the fovea.

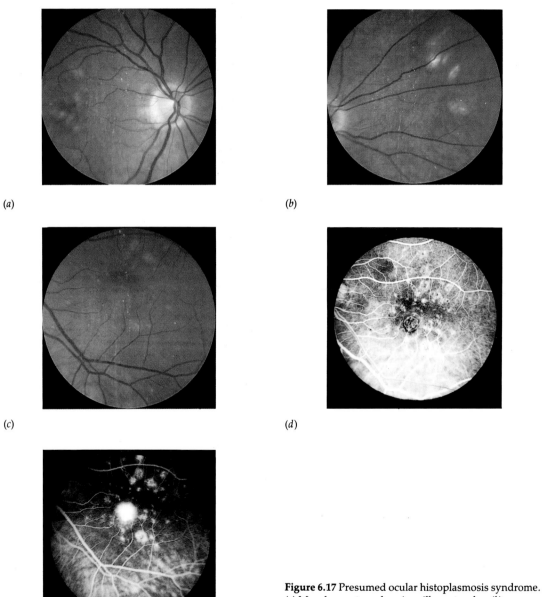

(a)

(b)

(c)

(d)

(e)

Figure 6.17 Presumed ocular histoplasmosis syndrome. (a) Macular spots and peripapillary atrophy. (b) Peripheral choroidal atrophic spots. (c) Disciform macular lesion. (d) and (e) Angiogram of (c) with subretinal new vessels

Pseudoxanthoma elasticum and angioid streaks

Angioid streaks of Bruch's membrane are found in pseudoxanthoma elasticum (PXE), Paget's disease, sickle cell disease, Ehlers–Danlos syndrome and sometimes idiopathically. Bruch's membrane becomes weakened by loss of elastin and calcium deposition. The resulting splits give the characteristic fundus appearance.

PXE is the most common cause of angioid streaks. It is usually dominantly inherited and gives rise to disorders in those tissues of the body with a high elastin content: the dermis of the neck, abdomen and flexor surface of the elbows becomes irregular and mottled (plucked chicken skin) (Figure 6.18), the aortic ring may become expanded leading to valvular incompetence and gastrointestinal bleeding can occur.

Clinical features   Initially the fundus may show only the signs of angioid streaks and vision is unaffected but neovascularization through a defect in Bruch's membrane often follows some years later (Figure 6.19). This may arise through a visible angioid streak but frequently originates from a microscopical break near the fovea which is not ophthalmoscopically visible.

Treatment   This is is usually unrewarding. Photocoagulation for new vessel complexes not underlying the fovea can be tried but because of the widespread nature of the process the result is often disappointing and further neovascularization occurs. Occasional therapeutic success can result however, and treatment may be worth trying for patients with severe metamorphopsia.

Best's disease (vitelliform dystrophy)

Best's disease is a dominantly inherited disorder usually affecting children in the first two decades of life. It may become manifest in middle age and in such cases the lesions are often multiple.

The condition is characterized by an accumulation of yellow material under the pigment epithelium at the posterior pole; the nature of this deposit is unknown.

Clinical features   Vision in the early stages of the process is only mildly affected in spite of an obviously visible yellow dome at the fovea. The overlying neuroretina is normal and is not elevated from the pigment epithelium (Figure 6.20). Sometimes the amorphous looking yellow material forms a pseudohypopyon and in the later stages often becomes irregular. This latter change is associated with the development of choroidal neovascularization through Bruch's membrane, at which time there is significant loss of central vision. Ultimately a fibrous disciform scar develops.

The electroretinogram is usually normal but the electro-oculogram is profoundly affected both in clinically affected patients and in carriers of the disease. In sporadically-affected middle-aged patients the EOG is often normal.

No treatment is available.

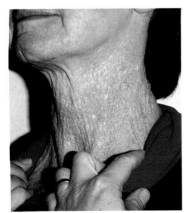

Figure 6.18 Skin of neck in pseudoxanthoma elasticum

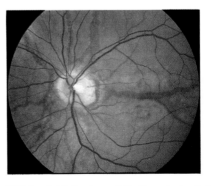

Figure 6.19 Angioid streaks and disciform lesion in PXE

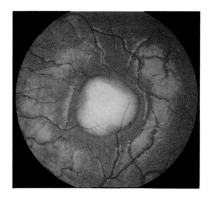

(a)

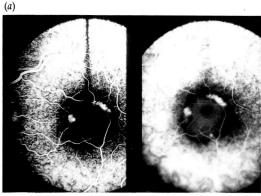

(b)

Figure 6.20 (a) Best's vitelliform dystrophy. Note early irregularity of the lesion on nasal and superior edges. (b) Angiogram of (a). Note only slight masking of the lesion and early neovascularization at the irregular edge

Choroidal ruptures

Ruptures of the posterior choroid develop as a result of blunt trauma. Immediately after injury haemorrhage under the pigment epithelium or neuroretina obscures the underlying rupture. The neuroretina is also often white from cloudy swelling of the axons of the ganglion cell layer (Berlin's oedema). As the acute process subsides the white linear ruptures become visible and they are often arcuate and concentric with the disc (Figure 6.21).

In addition to damage to the choroid, Bruch's membrane is also split and, if such dehiscences are close to the fovea, secondary neovascularization may follow (Figure 6.21). This can be a serious complication in an eye which had otherwise recovered good vision. Photocoagulation should be tried for those eccentric disciform lesions with subretinal fluid at the fovea and in whom there is demonstrable growth of the neovascular complex.

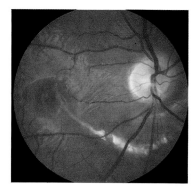

Figure 6.21 Choroidal rupture with neovascular membrane growing from the point nearest the fovea

Rare inherited causes of disciform lesions

Sorsby's pseudoinflammatory macular dystrophy is a dominantly inherited disorder becoming manifest in the fourth decade. After many years the pigment epithelium over a wide area becomes atrophic with severe loss of vision. Disciform lesions are common in these patients.

Polymorphous dystrophy is also dominantly inherited but patients show variable expression of the disease. Some have only mild pigment epithelial atrophy whereas others have marked posterior pole lesions often described incorrectly as macular colobomata. The disease begins in childhood.

Disciform degeneration has been described in a variety of photoreceptor degenerations. Retinitis pigmentosa, cone–rod dystrophy, cone dystrophy and Stargadt's disease have all been seen in association with macular choroidal neovascularization. Treatment is rarely possible but management is carried out on the lines of other forms of neovascular disciform degeneration.

Retinal vascular disease

Rarely cases of diabetic retinopathy and branch or central retinal vein occlusion may have a secondary disciform lesion. Such lesions tend to occur in the elderly who are subject to ageing macular degeneration and these associations may be by chance rather than causative.

Although treatment with photocoagulation can be considered the results are usually poor in view of the concurrent retinal vascular disease. It should be born in mind, however, that photocoagulation for a primary vascular disorder can induce a secondary disciform lesion from parafoveal damage to the pigment epithelium and Bruch's membrane.

Disciform lesions secondary to optic disc disease

Swelling of the optic disc is a recognized cause of peripapillar disciform lesions. Papilloedema and

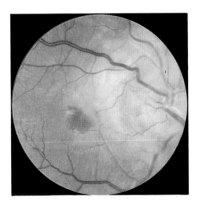

(a)

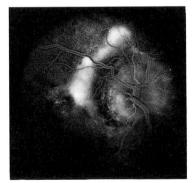

(b)

Figure 6.22 (*a*) Peripapillary disciform lesion with subretinal fluid extending to the fovea. (*b*) Angiogram of (*a*)

optic disc drusen have been implicated in this way but many peripapillary disciform lesions occur in the absence of clinically obvious disc swelling. It is presumed that choroidal neovascularization enters the subpigment epithelial space or subretinal space round the edge of Bruch's membrane where it terminates at the disc margin (Figure 6.22).

Peripapillary disciform lesions are less likely to grow and affect the fovea than those arising near the fovea. They can usually be watched by serial fluorescein angiography, and laser treatment is only necessary when the choroidal new vessels are demonstrated to be advancing towards the fovea. However, it should be remembered that in some cases peripapillary new vessels are capable of considerable growth and may also bleed. Careful review is usually required in the early stages.

Idiopathic disciform degeneration

In some cases spontaneous choroidal neovascularization occurs in an eye with no obvious underlying disease. Once the process begins it is impossible to know whether there was a small underlying area of atrophy or damage to Bruch's membrane present previously. A pre-existing lesion may explain some cases but it seems likely that there are a number of patients who develop disciform degeneration *de novo*. This may be the case with juvenile disciform degeneration (Figure 6.23) but when a child or teenager has neovascularization other family members must be examined to exclude inherited dystrophic conditions.

Disciform degeneration without overt neovascularization

Central serous retinopathy (CSR)

This common condition affects males more commonly than females (8:1) and occurs between the ages of 30 and 55 years with a maximum incidence at 42 years. It is usually a benign disease in Western countries but more severe in Orientals.

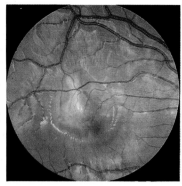

(a)

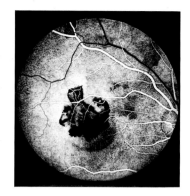

(b)

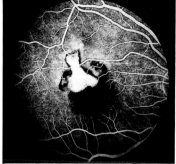

(c)

Figure 6.23 (*a*) Juvenile disciform degeneration in a girl of 13 years, VA 6/36. (*b*) and (*c*) Angiogram of (*a*).

Pathogenesis

Serous fluid accumulates in the subretinal space causing separation of the neuroretina from the pigment epithelium. A small cluster of pigment epithelial cells becomes defective leading to a break down of the outer blood–retinal barrier. Fluid from the extracellular space of the choroid passes through the defect and pools in the subretinal space. In most cases spontaneous healing and restoration of the outer blood–retinal barrier occurs, with subsequent absorption of the subretinal fluid, but in a few patients the pigment epithelium remains defective.

Although no systemic disease has a proven association with CSR it has been suggested that the incidence might be higher in patients with atopic diseases and in those of an anxious temperament.

Clinical features

The main symptoms of CSR are mild blurring of vision, micropsia, metamorphopsia and disturbances of colour vision. Objective visual acuity is often within normal limits especially if a small hypermetropic correction is used. Some patients have more serious loss of acuity but it is unusual for vision to be worse than 6/24. An Amsler chart will usually outline the area of vision affected by subretinal fluid.

The retina appears elevated on slit-lamp biomicroscopy (Figure 6.24) but sometimes care is needed to identify shallow subretinal fluid. The area of detachment almost invariably affects the fovea because symptoms are relatively mild and peripheral lesions do not disturb vision. In most cases the area of detachment is one or two disc diameters across but very rarely sub-total retinal

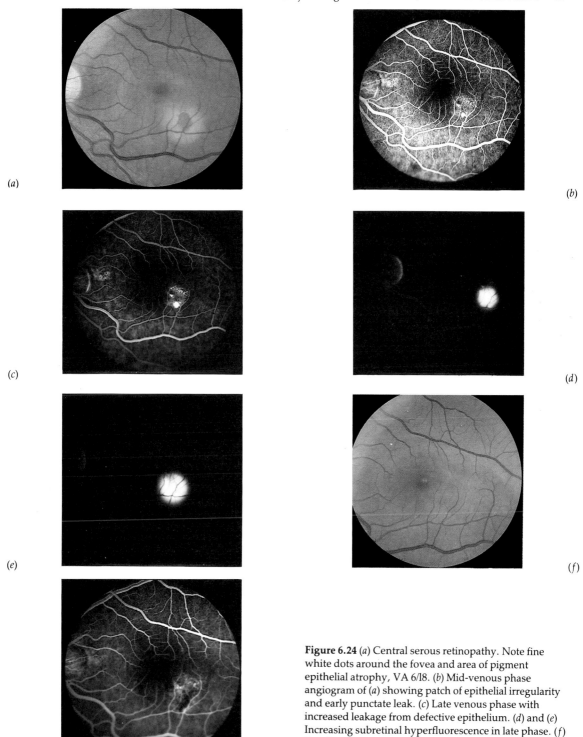

Figure 6.24 (*a*) Central serous retinopathy. Note fine white dots around the fovea and area of pigment epithelial atrophy, VA 6/18. (*b*) Mid-venous phase angiogram of (*a*) showing patch of epithelial irregularity and early punctate leak. (*c*) Late venous phase with increased leakage from defective epithelium. (*d*) and (*e*) Increasing subretinal hyperfluorescence in late phase. (*f*) Resolution of subretinal fluid after laser treatment, VA 6/9. (*g*) Angiogram of (*f*) confirming abolition of leakage

detachments can occur. A useful diagnostic sign is the presence of small white spots on the outer surface of the neuroretina. The pigment epithelium often shows patches of atrophy, especially at the point of leakage, and sometimes there is pigment epithelial irregularity in the fellow eye. A central serous punctate leak may also occur on the surface of a pigment epithelial detachment.

Fluorescein angiography

This can be helpful in confirming the diagnosis and pinpointing the leak. The area of outer blood–retinal barrier breakdown is outlined as a small punctate spot of dye beginning in the venous phase and gradually increasing in hyperfluorescence (Figure 6.24). Later in the run the dye diffuses outwards to fill the area of detachment and occasionally produces a typical 'smoke-stack' pattern. Care must be taken, especially in older patients, that the area of leakage is not in fact a small neovascular membrane and that the serous detachment is not a result of an early vascular disciform process.

Treatment

In the large majority of cases no active intervention is required and the patient can be reassured that resolution of the detachment will occur in 3–4 months from the onset. However, patients should be warned that in many cases the vision will not return completely to normal and that mild distortion and colour desaturation may persist.

Careful studies of laser photocoagulation for CSR have shown that the subretinal fluid absorbs more quickly following treatment, but there is little evidence to suggest that the final vision is better after photocoagulation compared with the natural outcome. For some patients CSR is a considerable handicap especially if fine binocular vision is required for their occupation. Such cases should be considered for laser treatment especially if the CSR persists for more than a few months. Also patients with progressive loss of acuity not correctable by hypermetropic lenses should be treated.

Laser photocoagulation is best carried out by one or two applications directly to the point of leakage demonstrable on fluorescein angiography; 200 µm, 0.1 second, gentle burns to give mild blanching of the pigment epithelium is sufficient to destroy the affected cells and allow adjacent cells to heal the blood–retinal barrier (Figure 6.24). Subretinal fluid absorbs within a few days and vision continues to improve for several weeks.

A minority of patients have persistence of subretinal fluid in spite of treatment. Multiple leaks and widespread atrophy of the pigment epithelium can also be encountered. In these instances CSR is a much less benign condition, often leading to permanent loss of central vision. Repeated laser treatment can be tried but is frequently ineffective.

Retinal pigment epithelial detachment

In the healthy state the pigment epithelium is adherent firmly to Bruch's membrane and cannot be easily separated. In the ageing eye this

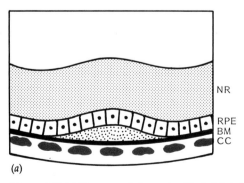
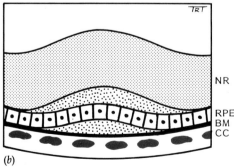

Figure 6.25 (*a*) Diagram of pigment epithelial detachment. (*b*) Diagram of pigment epithelial detachment with subretinal fluid. NR = neuroretina; RPE = pigment epithelium; BM = Bruch's membrane; CC = choriocapillaris

adhesion may become weakened and some patients develop elevation of the pigment epithelium.

Pathogenesis

Ageing changes in Bruch's membrane lead to thickening and disorganization of the collagen, lipid deposition and formation of drusen (see p. 55). In addition sometimes there is deposition of material in the basement membrane of the pigment epithelial cells (basal linear deposit). This combination of factors weakens the adhesion of the basement membrane to Bruch's membrane.

The pigment epithelium actively transports fluid from the neuroretina through Bruch's membrane to the choroid. It is likely that the increase in thickness and lipid deposition in Bruch's membrane make it relatively impermeable to water resulting in the pigment epithelium pumping itself off Bruch's membrane. Although this theory is not proven it does explain why an otherwise intact pigment epithelium separates from what is usually a firm bond to Bruch's membrane. Once the pigment epithelium becomes detached it usually remains elevated for prolonged periods of several years. In 50% of cases new vessels from the choriocapillaris invade the subpigment epithelial space and the process changes its character into a neovascular disciform lesion with subretinal fluid. In those cases in whom new vessels do not develop, the pigment epithelium may either remain intact or the outer blood–retinal barrier may become pervious, thus allowing fluid to collect in the subretinal space giving an avascular disciform lesion (Figure 6.25).

Clinical features

Pigment epithelial detachments cause similar symptoms to vascular disciform lesions but the visual disturbance tends to be milder when no subretinal fluid is present. Simple epithelial detachments, therefore, nearly always underlie the fovea because eccentric lesions are asymptomatic. Once subretinal fluid forms in the subretinal space symptoms become more pronounced with metamorphopsia and blurred vision.

Examination by slit-lamp biomicroscopy is the best method of identifying pigment epithelial detachments which can sometimes be difficult to observe by direct or indirect ophthalmoscopy. Identification is sometimes made easier by melanotic pigment figures on the elevated dome of epithelium and by subretinal fluid.

Closer examination of pigment epithelial detachments shows that different characteristics can be observed. Some show translucency of the subpigment epithelial fluid, which is easily seen on retroillumination, whereas others show marked turbidity from either lipid or blood in the subpigment epithelial space (Figures 6.26 and 6.27). The presence of blood indicates choroidal neovascularization. Subretinal lipid deposition can sometimes be seen and, although suggestive of the presence of new vessels, this is not invariably the case and may be simply an indication of the chronicity of the lesion.

Fluorescein angiography

This has allowed subclassification of pigment epithelial detachments into three types:

1. Early, even hyperfluorescence with dye beginning to fill the subretinal space in the capillary phase and gradually increasing in density (Figure 6.26).
2. Late, even hyperfluorescence with dye entering the detachment in the late venous phase (Figure 6.27).
3. Irregular filling with fluorescein showing high- or low-intensity spots within the detachment (Figure 6.28).

The early fluorescent type corresponds to the translucent detachments observable clinically. Delayed filling results from deposition of lipid under the pigment epithelium preventing rapid diffusion of fluorescein into the subpigment epithelial space. Irregular filling is from vascularized detachments with high spots from foci of new vessels and dark areas from lipid or blood.

Treatment

Laser photocoagulation remains controversial. A controlled study of photocoagulation for pigment epithelial detachments has only been carried out once and the results were not encouraging. Treatment resulted in loss of vision for some patients soon after photocoagulation whereas control patients as a group maintained better

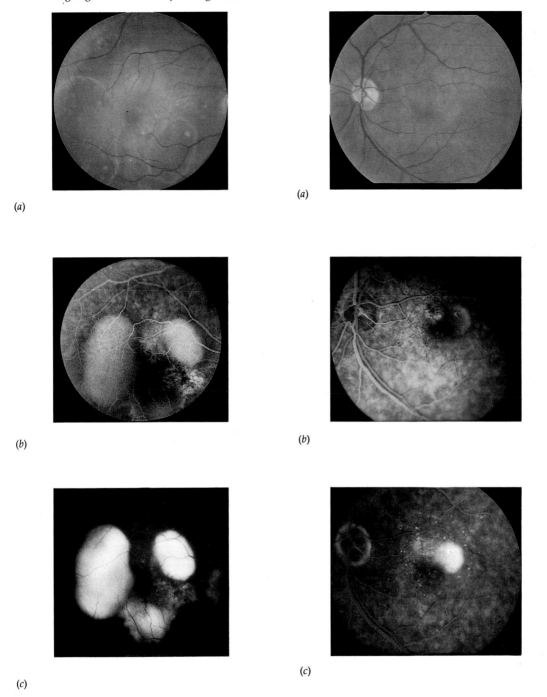

(a)

(b)

(c)

(a)

(b)

(c)

Figure 6.26 (*a*) Translucent pigment epithelial detachments. (*b*) and (*c*) Angiogram of (*a*) showing early even filling of the detachments with increasing fluorescence

Figure 6.27 (*a*) Pigment epithelial detachment adjacent and temporal to fovea. (*b*) and (*c*) Angiogram of (*a*) showing late filling after the venous phase. Note windowing of patchy RPE atrophy

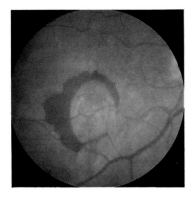

(a)

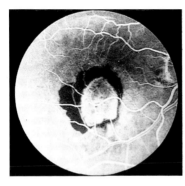

(b)

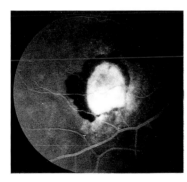

(c)

Figure 6.28 (*a*) Vascularized pigment epithelial detachment surrounded by haemorrhage. (*b*) and (*c*) Angiogram of (*a*). Note irregularity of hyperfluorescence lasting into later stage

vision for longer. However, the true picture is difficult to interpret because all types of pigment epithelial detachments were considered together and the long-term follow-up suggested that the ultimate visual prognosis may be as bad for untreated as for treated patients.

Treatment of translucent detachments usually leads to resolution of subpigment epithelial fluid and abolition of metamorphopsia, but it may be followed by epithelial atrophy and loss of visual acuity in some patients. Delayed filling detachments respond less readily to laser, often needing repeated treatment, and they have a higher risk of epithelial atrophy or neovascularization. Irregular filling detachments contain new vessels and should not be treated. Spontaneous resolution occurs in about 12% of cases and is normally in the translucent type of detachment.

If treatment by laser is carried out the patient should be warned that there is a 40% chance that it will fail and that some loss of acuity is a possibility. For patients in whom it is judged treatment should be attempted and who understand the risks, photocoagulation should be applied in a grid pattern. This allows the pigment epithelial cells to regenerate and subretinal fluid to absorb, possibly restoring better function. Applications of 200 μm causing mild blanching are scattered over the surface of the detachment with similar sized spaces between and avoiding the fovea. The best results are obtained in the translucent type of detachment which usually has a better natural prognosis.

Retinal pigment epithelial tears

Some cases of pigment epithelial detachments develop a tear around part of the edge of the dome of the epithelium.

Pathogenesis The mechanism of tearing of the pigment epithelium is disputed but two main theories have been suggested:

1. There is a pre-existing subretinal fibrovascular membrane which contracts and pulls on the elevated pigment epithelium causing a tear. Tearing of the pigment epithelium has been observed during photocoagulation of a choroidal neovascular disciform lesion and was thought to be due to contraction of the fibrovascular membrane.

2. The shearing forces around the elevation of the detachment are greatest at the edge where the dome joins the intact epithelium and mechanical force from cellular water transport tears the detachment rim. This would be particularly likely if the pigment epithelial cells separated from their basement membrane but this has not been conclusively shown to occur.

Clinical features The process of tearing of a pigment epithelial detachment is associated with marked loss of visual acuity. There may be pre-existing metamorphopsia from the underlying detachment but a considerable fall of vision is experienced after tearing.

The fundoscopic appearance is usually characteristic showing a dark irregular area of pigment epithelium with a sharply defined rolled-up edge of the retracted periphery of the tear. The bed of the tear is visible as a pink crescentic area of exposed Bruch's membrane and choriocapillaris (Figure 6.29). Subretinal fluid is invariably present in the early stage and haemorrhage is present in some cases.

After a few months the pigment epithelium repairs and the subretinal fluid absorbs leaving a shrunken mass of redundant pigment epithelium and fibrovascular tissue.

When a tear occurs in a previously observed pigment epithelial detachment, the detachment has usually had an irregular or turbid portion and a more highly elevated translucent portion. The tear occurs at the margin of the latter and it may be either spontaneous or follow photocoagulation.

Fluorescein angiography This shows irregular hypofluorescence in the area of rolled-up pigment epithelium and a neovascular membrane is sometimes seen. The exposed portion of the choriocapillaris fills with the normal choroidal flush and stains intensely in the later stages (Figure 6.29).

Treatment No treatment is currently available.

Occult neovascularization

Clinical features

Some patients present with typical symptoms of disciform degeneration and with subretinal fluid at the macula but do not have a visible neovascular complex on fluorescein angiography (Figure 6.30). These patients, in the absence of other causes of

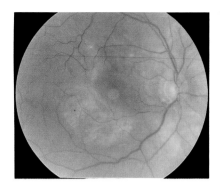

(a)

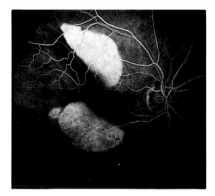

(b)

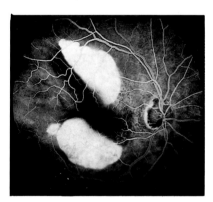

(c)

Figure 6.29 (a) Retinal pigment epithelial tear. Note dark edge of retracted pigment epithelium and lighter exposed choroid. (b) and (c) Angiogram of (a) with masking from the thick RPE and even hyperfluorescence of choriocapillaris

subretinal fluid and with signs of age-related degeneration such as drusen and pigment epithelial atrophy, are presumed to have occult neovascularization. Unlike typical vascular disciform disease the clinical course is often milder with preservation of reasonable visual acuity for many months or even a number of years.

Pathogenesis

Invasion of Bruch's membrane by new vessels from the choroid is common in the ageing eye (see p. 59). Where the overlying macular pigment epithelium is intact the new vesssels may remain latent and asymptomatic. In some cases the new vessels cause fluid to accumulate in the subretinal space but they do not become active proliferating vessel complexes.

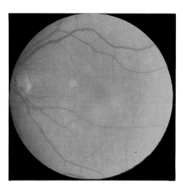

(a)

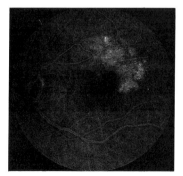

(b)

Figure 6.30 (a) Fundus with subretinal fluid at the macula from occult new vessels. (b) Late angiogram of (a) showing diffuse leakage of dye with no identifiable new vessels

Fluorescein angiography

This can be difficult to interpret particularly in the absence of stereo photographs. Multiple punctate spots of fluorescence appear relatively early in the run and then increase in staining becoming a confluent hyperfluorescent patch at the level of the pigment epithelium (Figure 6.30). Without stereo photographs to confirm the presence of subretinal fluid the angiographic picture resembles atrophy of the pigment epithelium and staining of drusen. The hyperfluorescence may occur either under the fovea or eccentrically.

Treatment

The principles of treatment by laser photocoagulation for overt neovascular membranes can be applied. Where new vessels affect the subfoveal pigment epithelium treatment should be withheld. When the fluorescence is parafoveal confluent photocoagulation can be applied over the whole area, similar to the treatment of identifiable new vessels (see p. 62).

Visual acuity usually remains at pretreatment levels but metamorphopsia resolves after absorption of subretinal fluid. The results of treatment are comparable with those of overt neovascularization but failure to obliterate the new vessels often leads to aggressive growth of neovascular membranes. It should also be remembered that the natural outcome is often better than in neovascular lesions and partial treatment should be avoided in case aggressive neovascularization is induced.

Further reading

BIRD, A. C. and GREY, R. H. B. (1979) Photocoagulation of disciform macular lesions with krypton laser. *British Journal of Ophthalmology*, **63**, 669–673

CASSWELL, A. G., KOHEN, D. and BIRD, A. C. (1985) Retinal pigment epithelial detachments in the elderly; classification and outcome. *British Journal of Ophthalmology*, **69**, 397–403

CHISHOLM, I. H. (1983) The recurrence of neovascularisation and late visual failure in senile disciform lesions. *Transactions of the Ophthalmological Society of the UK*, **103**, 354–359

COSCAS, G. and SOUBRANE, G. (1982) Photocoagulation des néovaisseaux sous rétiniens dans la dégénérescence maculaire sénile par le laser à argon: résultats de l'étude randomisée de 60 cas. *Bulletin Mémoire Société Français Ophthalmologie*, **88**, 102–105

DEUTMAN, A. F. and JANSEN, L. M. A. A. (1970) Dominantly inherited drusen of Bruch's membrane. *British Journal of Ophthalmology*, **54**, 373–382

DEUTMAN, A. F. and KOVACS, B. (1979) Argon laser treatment in complications of angioid streaks. *American Journal of Ophthalmology*, **88**, 12–17

FEENEY BURNS, L. and ELLERSIECK, M. R. (1985) Age related changes in the ultra structure of Bruch's membrane. *American Journal of Ophthalmology*, **100**, 686–697

FICKER, L., VAFIDIS, G., WHILE, A. and LEAVER, P. (1988) Long term follow up of a prospective trial of argon laser photocoagulation in the treatment of central serous retinopathy. *British Journal of Ophthalmology*, **72**, 829–834

GASS, J. D. M. (1967) The pathogenesis of disciform detachment of the neuroepithelium. *American Journal of Ophthalmology*, **63**, 573–586

GASS, J. D. M. (1973) Drusen and disciform detachment, macular detachment and degeneration. *Archives of Ophthalmology*, **90**, 206–217

GASS, J. D. M. (1987) *Stereoscopic Atlas of Macular Diseases*, 3rd edn., C. V. Mosby, New York

GELISKEN, O., HENDRIKSE, M. D. and DEUTMAN, A. F. (1988) A long-term follow-up study of laser coagulation of neovascular membranes in angioid streaks. *American Journal of Ophthalmology*, **105**, 299–303

GREGOR, Z., BIRD, A. C. and CHISHOLM, I. H. (1977) Senile disciform degeneration in the second eye. *British Journal of Ophthalmology*, **61**, 141–147

GREY, R. H. B., BIRD, A. C. and CHISHOLM, I. H. (1979) Senile disciform macular degeneration: features indicating suitability for photocoagulation. *British Journal of Ophthalmology*, **63**, 85–89

HILTON, G. F. (1975) Later serosanguineous detachment of the macula after traumatic choroidal rupture. *American Journal of Ophthalmology*, **79**, 991–1000

HOGAN, M. J. (1967) Bruch's membrane and disease of the macula. The role of elastic tissue and collagen. *Transactions of the Ophthalmological Society of the UK*, **87**, 113–161

HOSKIN, A., BIRD, A. C. and SEHMI, K. (1981) Tears of the detached retinal pigment epithelium. *British Journal of Ophthalmology*, **65**, 417–422

HOTCHKISS, M. L. and FINE, S. L. (1981) Pathological myopia and choroidal neovascularisation. *American Journal of Ophthalmology*, **91**, 177–183

KEIS, J. C. and BIRD, A. C. (1988) Juxtapapillary choroidal neovascularisation in older patients. *American Journal of Ophthalmology*, **105**, 11–19

KRILL, A. E. (1977) *Hereditary Retinal and Choroidal Diseases*, Vol. II, Harper and Row, New York

KRISHAN, N. R., CHANDRA, S. R. and STEVENS, T. S. (1985) Diagnosis and pathogenesis of retinal pigment epithelial tears. *American Journal of Ophthalmology*, **100**, 698–707

LEAVER, P. K. and WILLIAMS, C. (1979) Argon laser photocoagulation in the treatment of central serous retinopathy. *British Journal of Ophthalmology*, **63**, 674–677

MACULAR PHOTOCOAGULATION STUDY GROUP (1982) Argon laser photocoagulation for senile macular degeneration. Results of a randomised clinical trial. *Archives of Ophthalmology*, **100**, 912–918

MACULAR PHOTOCOAGULATION STUDY GROUP (1983) Argon laser photocoagulation for ocular histoplasmosis. Results of a randomized clinical trial. *Archives of Ophthalmology*, **101**, 1347–1357

MACULAR PHOTOCOAGULATION STUDY GROUP (1983) Argon laser photocoagulation for idiopathic neovascularisation. *Archives of Ophthalmology*, **101**, 1358–1361

MACULAR PHOTOCOAGULATION STUDY GROUP (1986) Recurrent choroidal neovascularisation after argon laser photocoagulation for neovascular maculopathy. *Archives of Ophthalmology*, **104**, 503–512

MACULAR PHOTOCOAGULATION STUDY GROUP (1986) Argon laser photocoagulation for neovascular maculopathy: Three-year results from radomised clinical trials. *Archives of Ophthalmology*, **104**, 694–701

MAGUIRE, P. and VINE, A. K. (1986) Geographic atrophy of the retinal pigment epithelium. *American Journal of Ophthalmology*, **102**, 621–625

MEREDITH, T. A., BRALEY, R. E. and AABERG, T. M. (1979) Natural history of serous detachments of the retinal pigment epithelium. *American Journal of Ophthalmology*, **88**, 643–651

MILLER, H., MILLER, B. and RYAN, S. J. (1985) Correlation of choroidal subretinal neovascularisation with fluorescein angiography. *American Journal of Ophthalmology*, **99**, 263–271

MOORFIELDS MACULAR STUDY GROUP (1982) Retinal pigment epithelial detachments in the elderly. A controlled trial of argon laser photocoagulation. *British Journal of Ophthalmology*, **66**, 1–16

MORSE, P. H. (1987) Decompensation of the retinal pigment epithelium and occult choroidal neovascularisation: indications for treatment. *Annals of Ophthalmology*, **19**, 276–279

ROBERTSON, D. H. (1986) Argon laser photocoagulation treatment in central serous chorioretinopathy. *Ophthalmology*, **93**, 972–974

SARKS, S. H. (1973) New vessel formation beneath the retinal pigment epithelium in senile eyes. *British Journal of Ophthalmology*, **57**, 951–965

SARKS, S. H. (1976) Ageing and degeneration in the macular region: a clinico-pathological study. *British Journal of Ophthalmology*, **60**, 324–341

SCHLAEGEL, T. F. (1977) *Ocular Histoplasmosis*, Grune and Stratton, New York

SHILLING, J. S. and BLACH, R. K. (1975) Prognosis and therapy of angioid streaks. *Transactions of the Ophthalmological Society of the UK*, **95**, 301–306

TEETERS, V. W. and BIRD, A. C. (1973) The development of neovascularisation of senile disciform degeneration. *American Journal of Ophthalmology*, **76**, 1–18

TEETERS, V. W. and BIRD, A. C. (1973) A clinical study of vascularity of senile disciform macular degeneration. *American Journal of Ophthalmology*, **75**, 523–565

7

Vascular malformations

Congenital malformations

Retinal telangiectasis (Leber's miliary aneurysms, Coats' disease)

Congenital vascular malformations are relatively uncommon, but retinal telangiectasis is the most often encountered. Typically it affects one eye of boys who present in the first decade of life, but girls can be affected and on some occasions both eyes may be involved. Histologically the vessels in the affected area are irregular and dilated, there is intraretinal and subretinal exudation with characteristic cholesterol crystals in the exudative material. Haemorrhages in the retina are sometimes present although they are not often observed on clinical examination. There is an unexplained association of retinal telangiectasis with retinitis pigmentosa.

Clinical features

The commonest forms of presentation are strabismus, leukocoria or reduced vision discovered at a routine school screening test. Generally, the younger the child presents, the more severe the disease and the most severe presentation is of a baby with leukocoria and total exudative retinal detachment (Figure 7.1). Examination under anaesthesia may be required to exclude other causes of leukocoria, particularly retinoblastoma. The grossly dilated retinal vasculature normally establishes the diagnosis but if there is doubt radiography or CT scanning may be needed.

In less severely affected cases vision is lost insidiously over a period of months or years and the child often presents with strabismus or having failed a school medical check. Fundoscopy reveals retinal exudation and dilatation of one or more areas of the capillary bed. The larger arterioles and venules are tortuous with irregular saccular dilatations (Figure 7.2).

Characteristically the retinal exudate affects the macula and also forms circinate deposits in the more peripheral retina around the areas of telangiectasia. The macula may be affected by exudate and oedema even though the posterior polar capillaries appear normal. When central exudates are seen in a fundus it is important to

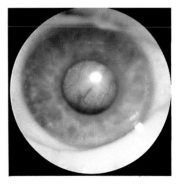

Figure 7.1 Leukocoria from advanced Coats' disease

81

examine the retinal periphery for vascular anomalies. In addition to exudate the macula may also be elevated by subretinal fluid (Figure 7.3) or by a fibrovascular scar (Figure 7.4).

Fluorescein angiography

This is not usually required to establish the diagnosis and is often not possible with small children. When performed it reveals widespread areas of retinal capillary dilatation and patchy capillary loss. The larger vessels are tortuous and dilated. The dye transit is rapid because of the high flow state and fluorescein readily leaks through both larger and smaller vessels (Figure 7.2).

Treatment

In mild cases in which there is no threat to the fovea by exudate deposition observation is the best course. If the fovea is about to be or already has become affected by increasing exudate, photocoagulation of the peripheral vascular defects is the treatment of choice. Small children require general anaesthesia for photocoagulation but for older children use of the argon laser can be attempted at an out patient clinic.

Direct photocoagulation of the major visible telangiectatic capillaries will lead to their regression and to clearance of the exudates. Several months should be allowed to elapse after each treatment because resolution is often slow (Figure 7.5).

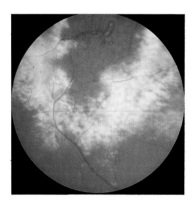

(a)

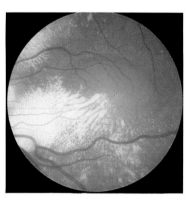

Figure 7.3 Macula of 14-year-old boy with parafoveal exudate and macular subretinal fluid from peripheral telangiectasia

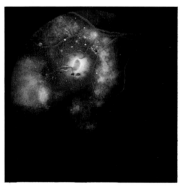

(b)
Figure 7.2 (a) Telangiectasia of retinal vessels with marked exudation in a boy aged 12 years. (b) Angiogram of (a) showing dilated vessels and fluorescein leakage

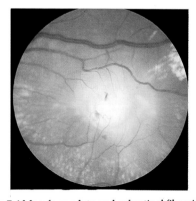

Figure 7.4 Macula exudate and subretinal fibrosis from telangiectasia in a 13-year-old girl

Cryotherapy can be used as an alternative method of treatment and can be useful in young children and for telangiectasia in the far retinal periphery. Care must be exercised to prevent secondary retinal detachment and multiple treatment sessions may be required for extensive disease.

Once the macula is affected by a fibrovascular scar, treatment will not restore visual acuity. However, it may be necessary to prevent progressive massive exudation and loss of useful peripheral visual field. Retinal detachment from telangiectasia is difficult to treat and is usually unrewarding, particularly when the fellow eye is normal. In order to reattach the retina it is usually necessary to perform a vitrectomy, gas tamponade and intraoperative endo-photocoagulation.

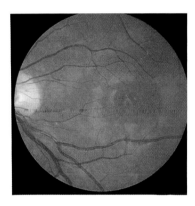

Figure 7.5 Macula of case in Figure 7.3, 2 years after peripheral laser treatment directly to visible telangiectatic vessels

Von Hippel–Lindau disease (angiomatosis retinae)

Von Hippel–Lindau disease, along with von Recklinghausen's disease, Sturge–Weber syndrome and tuberous sclerosis, forms part of the rare group of disorders known as the phakomatoses (birthmarks). Only von Hippel–Lindau and Sturge–Weber disease develop vascular anomalies in the fundus, whereas von Recklinghausen and tuberous sclerosis form astrocytomas. All these conditions share in common autosomal dominant inheritance with variable penetrance.

Von Hippel–Lindau disease is characterized by retinal angiomatous tumours. The tumours consist of endothelial and glial cells which form multiple vascular channels. The tumours can arise in any area of the retina and fresh lesions may develop in previously unaffected parts of the retina at any time in the first two or three decades of life.

As well as ocular disease there is a strong tendency towards cerebellar haemangioblastoma and also polycystic lesions in the abdominal viscera or renal carcinoma. The systemic manifestations, particularly the intracranial tumours, carry a poor prognosis and intracranial haemorrhages or effects from a space-occupying lesion in the posterior fossa are often fatal.

Clinical features

In the early stages angiomatous tumours may be asymptomatic. In time secondary effects from exudation, haemorrhage or retinal detachment reduce vision.

Early lesions consist of pink elevated masses in the peripheral retina. Invariably vitreous condensations inserting into the tumour produce vitreoretinal traction, although this is not always of clinical significance. One of the typical hallmarks of the disease is the pronounced dilatation of the feeding arteriole and draining venule supplying the tumours (Figure 7.6). Because the angiomas have numerous vascular channels there is a high blood flow through the mass causing this marked vessel dilatation.

Once tumours have started there is gradual enlargement of the mass and a high risk of secondary retinal detachment either from subretinal exudation or from vitreoretinal traction.

Fluorescein angiography is not usually necessary in establishing the diagnosis but, if performed, reveals gross dye leakage (Figure 7.6). Serial colour photography can be useful in documenting tumour growth.

Treatment

Photocoagulation or cryotherapy are the treatments of choice. Laser photocoagulation is difficult in children and often requires repeated sessions to shrink the tumour but is a good method for adults. Xenon photocoagulation is the traditional method of treatment and remains

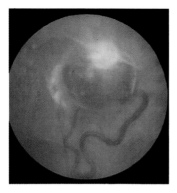

(a)

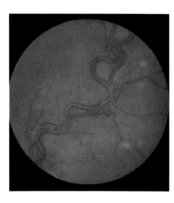

(b)

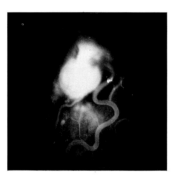

(c)

Figure 7.6 (a) Angioma of peripheral retina. (b) Dilated retinal vessels supplying the tumour. (c) Angiogram of (a) with marked leakage from the shunting capillary mass

useful in children when general anaesthesia is needed or in cases unresponsive to laser.

Cryotherapy is helpful for peripheral or for large tumours and can be applied either in a single or triple freeze technique. However, care must be exercised because vigorous treatment can lead to secondary retinal detachment with a poor visual prognosis. If multiple tumours are present it is safer to divide the treatment into a number of sessions.

After successful treatment long-term follow-up is necessary in case fresh angiomas develop in new sites of previously unaffected retina.

Juxtapapillary haemangioma

Juxtapapillary haemangioma of the retina is a rare condition producing a capillary anomaly in the neuroretina close to the optic nerve head. These malformations have a tendency to produce serous detachment and because of their location the macula is often affected. Treatment by photo-coagulation may be inadvisable when the tumour is in the papillomacular bundle because destruction of the angioma causes neuroretinal damage.

Sturge–Weber syndrome

Sturge–Weber syndrome consists of haemangiomatous malformations of the face and meninges. The most common ocular disease is congenital glaucoma (buphthalmos) but a diffuse angioma of the choroid may also be present. Dominant inheritance has been found but most cases appear to be isolated phenomena.

Histology of the angiomatous defects shows them to be cavernous capillary malformations occurring in the trigeminal distribution of the skin of the face, leptomeninges and buccal mucosa.

Clinical features

The most prominent feature of the syndrome is a facial angioma (port-wine stain or naevus flammeus) which, unlike a capillary haemangioma (strawberry naevus), does not disappear during the first few years of life. The affected skin is often hypertrophic (Figure 7.7).

Forty per cent of cases have buphthalmos and this is particularly common if the angioma involves the upper eyelid.

Choroidal involvement is much less common and is often asymptomatic. Typically large areas of the choroid show a diffuse dark redness when compared with normal parts of the fundus or to the fellow eye. The malformation is usually flat though may contain thickened areas and, therefore, appears different from the acquired localized form of choroidal haemangioma in adults (see p. 90). Serous retinal detachment may occur with accompanying loss of vision and it has been suggested this is more frequent in those malformations with thickening of the choroid.

The intracranial meningeal malformation is often silent but fits or hemiplegia can result. An X-ray of the skull may show typical parallel linear patterns of calcification in the vessel walls of the angioma.

Treatment

The traditional treatment for the skin has been to disguise the prominent facial defect with special cosmetics which can be highly effective. Argon laser photocoagulation to the skin has been used to occlude the vascular channels with considerable improvement in some cases but the treatment is time consuming, involving multiple sessions, and is not always beneficial.

The choroidal angioma does not require treatment unless exudative detachment of the retina is present. Unfortunately this type of angioma is widespread and difficult to photocoagulate adequately unless localized areas of leakage can be demonstrated on fluorescein angiography. In such cases argon or xenon photocoagulation to the leaking areas should be tried. Recently, with the newer techniques of localized radiotherapy, external radiation has been shown to reattach the retina but whether long-term benefit accrues has not yet been determined. Radiation damage to anterior or posterior segment structures from external radiation may be found to limit the long-term results.

Cavernous haemangioma of the retina

This rare developmental abnormality affects the retinal capillaries, usually in the periphery, but occasionally at the macula or optic disc. The defect appears to be caused by saccular dilatations arising from the capillary walls. Although the dilatations are filled with blood they are not in the mainstream of the circulation and, therefore, have slow blood flow, unlike retinal telangiectasis which shows rapid flow. There may also be accompanying cavernous haemangiomata of the cerebral cortex which can lead to fits or subarachnoid haemorrhages.

Clinical features

Ocular cavernous haemangioma is a benign condition producing little in the way of symptoms and is often discovered as a chance finding. Sometimes the angiomas bleed causing floaters from minor vitreous haemorrhages.

The fundus appearance is of a cluster of aneurysms affecting an area of the retina with or without overlying vitreous haemorrhage (Figure 7.8). Initial examination may be confused with retinal telangiectasis but the lesion is usually more circumscribed, the larger retinal vessels are not affected and there is no exudation from leaking capillaries.

Fluorescein angiography

This can be helpful in establishing the true diagnosis and differentiating cavernous haemangioma from telangiectasis. The flow through the

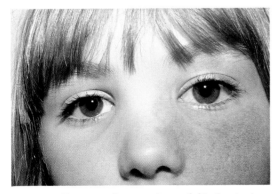

Figure 7.7 Cavernous haemangioma of skin (port-wine stain)

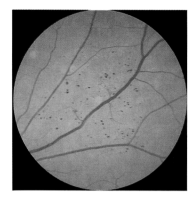

(a)

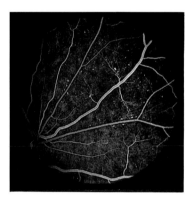

(b)

(c)

Figure 7.8 (*a*) Cavernous retinal haemangioma. (*b*)
Angiogram of (*a*). Note slow filling of malformation
unlike microaneurysm or telangiectasia. (*c*) Late phase of
cavernous haemangioma. Note lack of dye leakage and
long persistence of hyperfluorescence

saccular dilatations is slow and dye enters the
aneurysms late in the run. In addition typical fluid
levels may be seen as the sluggish blood cells
sediment causing masking of the lower half of the
aneurysm (Figure 7.8).

Treatment

Treatment is not required as vision is not
threatened unless recurrent vitreous haemorrhages occur. Photocoagulation of the angioma by
argon laser is effective in preventing further
haemorrhage.

Racemose angioma

Racemose angioma of the retina is a rare disorder
resulting from abnormal arterio-venous communications during the development of the retinal
circulation. Differing degrees of vascular involvement can be found. The abnormality may be either
confined to the retina or may extend posteriorly to
affect the optic nerve and midbrain (Wyburn–
Mason syndrome).

Clinical features

The fundal appearance of racemose angioma is
characteristic. There is massive dilatation of the
affected retinal vessels and arterialization of the
vein walls from the high blood flow (Figure 7.9).
The only other condition that is likely to cause
confusion is angiomatosis retinae with large feeder
vessels supplying the angioma; careful viewing of
the peripheral retina easily distinguishes the two
conditions.

Although racemose angioma does not change
rapidly, an increase in the vessel size can occur
over a period of years. If the optic nerve head is
affected the axons are compressed and vision is
gradually lost. Involvement of the optic chiasm by
the enlarged vessels can lead to optic nerve
compression and field loss on the opposite side.
Arteriography will then be required to find the
extent of the lesion and neurosurgical advice
should be sought.

Fluorescein angiography

This demonstrates the arterio-venous communications in the early stages of the dye transit. The high flow often produces multiple laminations in the venous circulation (Figure 7.9b).

Treatment

No treatment is available for the ophthalmic manifestations of the disease.

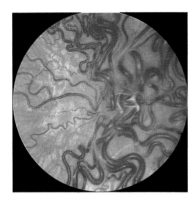

(a)

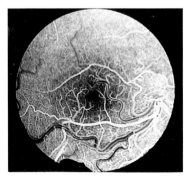

(b)

Figure 7.9 (*a*) Large racemose retinal angioma. (*b*) Angiogram of mild racemose angioma showing trilaminar flow in inferior veins

Acquired malformations

Retinal telangiectasis

Telangiectasis of retinal capillaries can present at any time of life and in a young adult it can be difficult to be certain whether the origin of the vascular defect is congenital or acquired. However, there is a group of patients in whom symptoms develop later in life and these cases are probably truly acquired telangiectasis. There is a preponderance of male patients and the condition is often unilateral but females can be affected or both eyes involved.

Clinical features

Retinal telangiectasis remains asymptomatic unless decompensation of the capillary walls occurs causing breakdown of the blood–retinal barrier. The fovea then becomes affected with exudate or oedema and patients are aware of a mild blurring and distortion of vision. Haemorrhage sometimes occurs giving a more acute disturbance of vision but acuity is usually 6/12 or better when first examined.

Ophthalmoscopy reveals the capillary disturbance and most often it is on the temporal side of the fovea. The signs are variable ranging from minimal disturbance, sometimes with a single microaneurysm, to scattered exudates, a few dot haemorrhages and foveal oedema (Figure 7.10).

Fluorescein angiography confirms the diagnosis and outlines the dilated parafoveal leaking capillaries. Some cases have a mild capillary loss (Figure 7.10). If the abnormality is circumscribed and lies above or below the fovea, the angiogram may resemble a small branch vein occlusion but the dilated capillary bed is not based on a venous tributary and the two disorders can usually be differentiated.

Treatment

Treatment is often not required as visual acuity remains normal for prolonged periods. If vision deteriorates over a period of several weeks or months, laser photocoagulation should be considered but care must be exercised during treatment as the leaking vessels are usually close to the fovea.

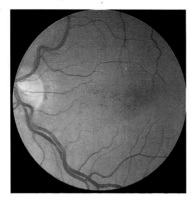

(a)

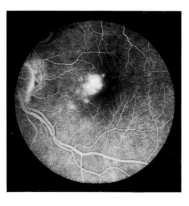

(b)

Treatment scotomata are common and can be as annoying to the patient as the original visual disturbance. When laser treatment is indicated it is advisable to use 100 μm applications producing a gentle reaction. Only the dilated vessels farthest from the fovea are treated first as this may be sufficient to reverse the exudate and oedema and cause the least obvious treatment scotoma. If this is unsuccessful, closer treatment can be tried provided due explanation is given to the patient.

Retinal macroaneurysm

This relatively common vascular disorder of the retinal circulation is an acquired lesion, usually in the elderly and in those with generalized vascular disease. However, it can sometimes be found in the absence of any antecedent cause. Either sex may be affected but there is a preponderance of females, and the lesions may be single or multiple, unilateral or bilateral.

Macroaneurysms arise from the larger arterioles in the posterior fundus and are often found on the second-order vessels. Because of the high incidence of essential hypertension and other cardiovascular defects macroaneurysms are probably a manifestation of generalized vascular disease. In particular, cerebrovascular accidents are common and similar aneurysmal dilatations have been found in the cerebral circulation.

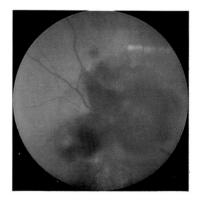

(c)

Figure 7.10 (a) Acquired retinal telangiectasia in a 64-year-old woman. (b) and (c) Angiogram of (a), showing loss of inner blood–retinal barrier

Figure 7.11 Acute haemorrhage from macroaneurysm with vitreous, pre, intra and subretinal blood

Clinical features

Macroaneurysms tend to fall into two clinical groups: those with an acute haemorrhagic episode or those with chronic exudation.

Patients with the acute form present with sudden loss or disturbance of vision resulting from rupture of the aneurysm. Blood leaks at relatively high arteriolar pressure and can, therefore, be extensive if the rupture in the vessel wall is large. Haemorrhage is found within the neuroretina, in the subretinal space and in the vitreous or subhyaloid space (Figure 7.11). Massive vitreous haemorrhage can reduce vision profoundly and this diagnosis should always be considered in patients presenting with sudden vitreous haemorrhage.

Fundoscopy often shows the retinal arteriole

beyond the aneurysm is of small calibre and it may even be occluded. A retinal branch vein occlusion may also be seen distal to the aneurysm.

Chronic exudative macroaneurysms present with progressive loss of central acuity from exudate deposition at the fovea. In most conditions exudates take many weeks or months to become deposited heavily but with a macroaneurysm gross deposits can build up over a much shorter period.

Unlike microaneurysms, macroaneurysms do not appear as red dots but as white or grey round lesions close to or directly over a retinal arteriole lying within the neuroretina. Because of the focal leakage the aneurysm is often in the centre of a surrounding haemorrhage or circinate exudate (Figure 7.12).

Fluorescein angiography can be helpful in

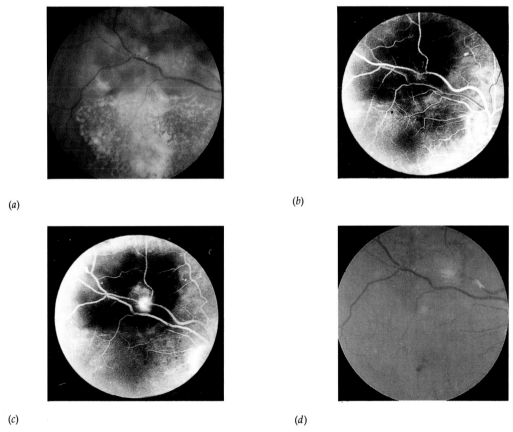

(a)

(b)

(c)

(d)

Figure 7.12 (*a*) Macroaneurysm of superotemporal arteriole producing gross macular exudation. (*b*) and (*c*) Angiogram of (*a*) with slow increase of hyperfluorescence from macroaneurysm. (*d*) Resolution of exudate 1 year after laser treatment

identifying the aneurysms, particularly if a branch vein occlusion is present, which may distract attention from the aneurysm itself. Typically the aneurysm is hypofluorescent in the early stages of the dye transit but leaks increasingly in the later stages (Figure 7.12). If the aneurysm is sclerosed or filled with blood clot there may be little filling with fluorescein. Evidence of branch retinal arteriolar or venular occlusion will be seen in those cases in which such an event has accompanied the macroaneurysm.

Treatment

Acute haemorrhagic decompensation of a macroaneurysm rarely requires active treatment. After the bleeding episode the aneurysm often hyalinizes and once the haemorrhage has absorbed the condition resolves. Vision usually returns to near normal levels unless the fovea has been seriously affected by haemorrhage or unless there has been concurrent venous obstruction.

Dense vitreous haemorrhage may require vitrectomy if spontaneous clearing does not occur after some months. However, the condition is usually uniocular and patients can be elderly and infirm from arteriosclerosis which may contraindicate general anaesthesia.

Chronic exudative macroaneurysms should be observed closely. If exudate or oedema affects the fovea, laser photocoagulation should be undertaken before acuity is severely reduced and it should be remembered that exudation may occur surprisingly quickly.

Photocoagulation with 200 μm spots around the aneurysm to produce a gentle reaction in the pigment epithelium is usually enough to prevent further leakage and reverses exudate deposition (Figure 7.12). Direct gentle treatment over the surface of the macroaneurysm can also be used with good effect but heavy photocoagulation should be avoided in case of aneurysmal rupture leading to severe haemorrhage.

Choroidal haemangioma

Unlike the choroidal haemangioma associated with Sturge–Weber syndrome, acquired haemangiomas are localized choroidal tumours which affect adults of middle age. These cavernous malformations probably develop earlier in life but only become diagnosed after the development of secondary retinal changes. Histologically they are composed of dilated venous channels with pigment disturbance and degeneration of the overlying retinal pigment epithelium.

Clinical features

The most common reason for presentation is the development of mild blurring and distortion of vision, not unlike patients with central serous retinopathy. The tumour itself rarely causes symptoms but the secondary changes of the overlying pigment epithelium lead to chronic subretinal fluid accumulation and foveal elevation from breakdown of the outer blood–retinal barrier.

Ophthalmoscopically, small choroidal haemangiomas can be difficult to identify but careful observation with the binocular indirect ophthalmoscope usually reveals the elevated choroidal mass. The angioma often has a slight orange colour with a mottled or linear pattern within it (Figure 7.13). Pigmentary changes on the overlying pigment epithelium can be helpful in highlighting the affected area. Subretinal fluid separating the neuroretina from the tumour is the rule with symptomatic lesions and this usually reaches the fovea but may be restricted to the area of the angioma for many years. The condition has to be differentiated from other causes of subretinal fluid at the macula, particularly choroidal neovascularization and central serous retinopathy and also from other choroidal masses such as melanoma, secondary tumours and choroidal osteoma.

Two investigations helpful in establishing the diagnosis are ultrasonography and fluorescein angiography. Ultrasonography shows very high reflectivity which helps to differentiate it from other fundus lesions, with the exception of osteoma of the choroid.

Fluorescein angiography demonstrates a variable pattern but often there is early rapid filling of the tumour and considerable fluorescence present before the retinal circulation fills (Figure 7.13). The later stages of the angiogram show intense hyperfluorescence with a mottled lobular pattern. Caution should be exercised in differentiating between a choroidal haemangioma and a choroidal melanoma on angiographic evidence alone as melanomas can be vascular and fill rapidly with dye.

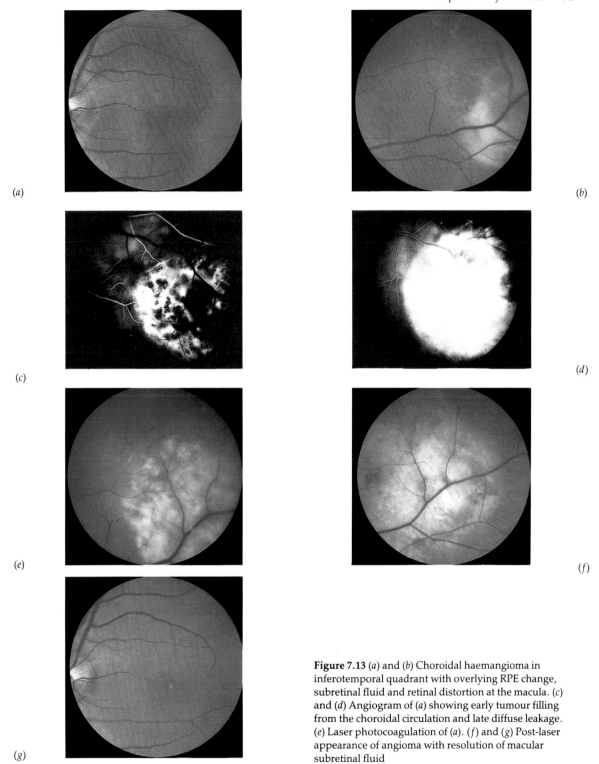

(a)

(b)

(c)

(d)

(e)

(f)

(g)

Figure 7.13 (*a*) and (*b*) Choroidal haemangioma in inferotemporal quadrant with overlying RPE change, subretinal fluid and retinal distortion at the macula. (*c*) and (*d*) Angiogram of (*a*) showing early tumour filling from the choroidal circulation and late diffuse leakage. (*e*) Laser photocoagulation of (*a*). (*f*) and (*g*) Post-laser appearance of angioma with resolution of macular subretinal fluid

Treatment

Treatment of choroidal haemangioma by photocoagulation is based on the principle of trying to absorb the subretinal fluid and not on trying to eradicate the tumour itself. The haemangioma is benign but produces visual loss from failure of the pigment epithelium to maintain the outer blood retinal barrier.

Contiguous 500 μm laser applications over the surface of the haemangioma sufficient to produce moderate blanching should be given (Figure 7.13). After several weeks, if there has not been adequate response, the treatment should be repeated and multiple retreatments are sometimes necessary.

It is usually adequate to resolve the submacular fluid as complete resolution of all subretinal fluid over the angioma is not always possible. Patients presenting with subretinal fluid confined over the tumour do not usually require treatment unless the fluid can be seen to advance towards the fovea.

If laser treatment fails xenon arc or triple freeze cryotherapy are alternative methods of therapy. Care has to be exercised when the angioma is close to the disc or the macula to prevent serious reduction of vision from the treatment.

Further reading

ABDEL-KHALEK, M. N. and RICHARDSON, J. (1986) Retinal macroaneurysm: natural history and guidelines for treatment. *British Journal of Ophthalmology*, **70**, 2–11

ARCHER, D. B., DEUTMAN, A., ERNEST, T. J. and KRILL, A. E. (1973) Arteriovenous communications of the retina. *American Journal of Ophthalmology*, **00**, 224–241

CASSWELL, A. G., CHAINE, G., RUSH, P. and BIRD, A. C. (1986) Paramacular telangiectasia. *Transactions of the Ophthalmological Society of the UK*, **105**, 683–692

CLEARY, P. E., KOHNER, E. M., HAMILTON, A. M. and BIRD, A. C. (1975) Retinal macroaneurysms. *British Journal of Ophthalmology*, **59**, 355–361

DUANE, T. D. Vascular anomalies. *Clinical Ophthalmology*, Vol. III, Chapter 22, Harper and Row, New York

DUANE, T. D. Phakomatoses. In *Clinical Ophthalmology*, Vol. V, Chapter 36, Harper and Row, New York

GASS, J. D. M. (1971) Cavernous haemangioma of the retina: a neuro-oculocutaneous syndrome. *American Journal of Ophthalmology*, **71**, 799–814

GASS, J. D. M. (1987) *Stereoscopic Atlas of Macular Diseases*, 3rd edn., C. V. Mosby, New York

GASS, J. D. and OYAKAWA, R. T. (1982) Idiopathic juxtafoveolar retinal telangiectasia. *Archives of Ophthalmology*, **100**, 796–780

GOLDBERG, M. F. and DUKE, J. R. (1968) Von Hippel–Lindau disease. *American Journal of Ophthalmology*, **66**, 693–705

KRILL, A. E. (1977) *Hereditary Retinal and Choroidal Diseases*, Vol. II, Harper and Row, New York

LAVIN, M. J., MARSH, R. J., PEART, S. and REHMAN, A. (1987) Retinal arterial macroaneurysms: a retrospective study of 40 patients. *British Journal of Ophthalmology*, **71**, 817–825

MESSMER, E., LAQUA, H., WESSING, A., et al. (1983) Nine cases of carvernous haemangioma of the retina. *American Journal of Ophthalmology*, **95**, 383–390

NORTON, E. W. D. and GUTMAN, F. (1967) Fluorescein angiography and haemangiomas of the choroid. *Archives of Ophthalmology*, **78**, 121–125

RIDLEY, M. E., SHIELDS, J. A., BROWN, G. C. and TASMAN, W. (1982) Coats' disease. Evaluation of management. *Ophthalmology*, **89**, 1381–1387

SPENCER, W. H. (1985) Congenital variations and anomalies. In *Ophthalmic Pathology*, Vol. II, Chapter 8, W. B. Saunders, Philadelphia

TARKKANEN, A. and LAATIKAINEN, L. (1983) Coats' disease: clinical angiographic, histopathological findings and clinical management. *British Journal of Ophthalmology*, **67**, 766–776

8

Retinal vasculitis and related disorders

There are a number of conditions causing systemic or ocular inflammation in which the retinal vasculature is involved as part of the disease process. In some cases, this is a secondary phenomenon following a generalized uveitis but in others retinal vascular changes occur as part of the primary disease process.

Idiopathic retinal vasculitis

In many patients presenting with inflammatory signs in the posterior segment, no underlying systemic cause can be identified in spite of extensive investigation. Retinal vasculitis and posterior uveitis may occur together as in sarcoidosis, toxoplasmosis or birdshot chorioretinopathy but inflammation of retinal vessels may also be seen in the absence of uveitis such as accompanying demyelinating diseases. The pathogenesis of the vessel wall changes is not well understood but it is likely that immune mechanisms are responsible. Some patients with idiopathic retinal vasculitis have circulating immune complexes and antibodies to retinal S antigen but whether this is the cause or effect of vasculitis is not known. Immune complexes and complement abnormalities are also features of systemic lupus erythematosus (SLE) which is a known cause of retinal vasculitis.

Abnormalities of cellular immunity have also been recognized in some conditions which are capable of producing retinal vasculitis, such as sarcoidosis, and autoantibodies can be a feature of systemic lupus erythematosus and Behçet's dis-

ease. Sensitization to retinal S antigen has been postulated as a cause of birdshot chorioretinopathy but it is unlikely that this is the mechanism in all types of vasculitis in the absence of outer retinal or choroidal disease. Conceivably such a mechanism could be implicated in the vasculitis observed in some patients with retinitis pigmentosa. Genetic susceptibility to retinal vasculitis may be important and an increased likelihood of carrying HLA-DR4 has been found and HLA-A29 is found in 96% of patients with birdshot choroidopathy.

The role of tuberculosis producing retinal vasculitis has been discussed on page 49 in conjunction with Eales disease, but active or old tuberculosis should be considered in all patients with vasculitis. In spite of careful investigation into systemic causes of vasculitis many patients have no underlying identifiable disease and until more is known about the aetiology of such cases they continue to be diagnosed as idiopathic vasculitis.

Clinical features

The clinical features of retinal vasculitis may affect both the arterial and venous sides of the circulation but usually the latter predominate. The peripheral fundus shows venous irregularities with perivascular sheathing (Figure 8.1). Scattered punctate haemorrhages are usually present but may be few in number. Cotton wool spots and arterial sheathing are sometimes present and in more severe cases peripheral vascular closure may occur leading to areas of peripheral neovascularization. In some cases new vessels may occur on the optic disc (Figure 8.2). Some degree of vitreous cellular infiltration is invariably present during active periods of the disease.

The clinical course of retinal vasculitis varies from mild floaters to severe visual loss. It is often protracted with episodes of activity and in some the outlook for vision without treatment is poor. In mild cases vision is well maintained but in more severe cases the disease continues low-grade activity for many years producing cataracts, chronic macular oedema, optic atrophy and vitreous haemorrhage from vasoproliferation.

Investigations

Investigation of retinal vasculitis should include screening for underlying immunological abnormalities and recognized specific causes of vasculitis such as sarcoidosis, tuberculosis, collagen disorders, multiple sclerosis, syphilis and Behçet's disease. It should be remembered that ocular ischaemia may present with a picture similar to vasculitis and investigation should be carried out for carotid artery obstruction and Takayasu's disease.

Fluorescein angiography is of limited help in the diagnosis of retinal vasculitis but can be useful in identifying macular oedema and assessing the response to treatment.

Treatment

Treatment is required when vision is seriously threatened. The major causes of loss of vision are chronic macular oedema, cataract and vitreous haemorrhage from peripheral or optic disc neovascularization.

Severe vasculitis or macular oedema causing visual loss should be treated with systemic steroids. Initially high doses are used to quieten the process, thereafter reducing to the lowest dose compatible with keeping the vasculitis to minimal activity. Because the disease has a protracted course, long-term steroid dosage may be required and it is, therefore, important to exclude active

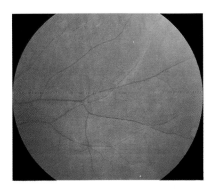

(a)

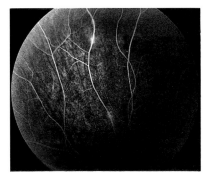

(b)

Figure 8.1 (*a*) Retinal vasculitis in temporal periphery of left eye showing sheathing and perivascular infiltration; (*b*) fluorescein angiogram of superior fundus of the same eye with focal staining of vessel walls

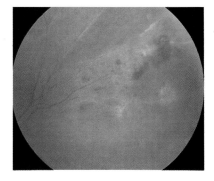

Figure 8.2 Peripheral neovascularization following vasculitis

tuberculosis. Acute exacerbations may require depot posterior sub-Tenon's or orbital floor steroid injections.

If the disease responds poorly to steroids, or if excessive dosage is needed with the accompanying risks of serious complications, immunosuppressive drugs can be used either instead of steroids or in combination. Chlorambucil or azathioprine are the most commonly used alternatives and are often better tolerated than steroids. Cyclosporin is being used increasingly as an alternative. When these drugs are used regular blood screening for bone marrow suppression must be performed and risks of infection or malignancy explained to the patient.

Sarcoidosis

Sarcoidosis is a non-caseating granulomatous disease mainly affecting the lungs, abdominal viscera, lymph nodes, skin and eyes. It is the commonest identifiable cause of retinal vasculitis and some form of ocular or orbital manifestation is present in about 40% of patients with the disease.

Clinical features

The main ocular manifestations are uveitis, lacrimal gland inflammation, and conjunctival infiltration but optic nerve infiltration, retinal vasculitis and central nervous system or meningeal disease may also occur.

The typical signs of posterior segment sarcoidosis are vitreous cells, so-called candle wax droppings on the retinal surface, dense infiltrations in the inferior vitreous gel, multiple choroidal granulomata, perivenous sheathing and irregularity of the retinal veins, scattered punctate retinal haemorrhages and macular oedema (Figure 8.3). When retinal vasculitis is severe there may be peripheral vascular closure and secondary retinal neovascularization from ischaemia.

Investigations

Investigations helpful in establishing the diagnosis of sarcoidosis include a chest X-ray for signs of

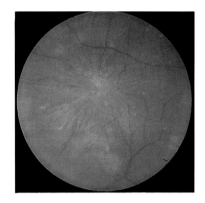

(a)

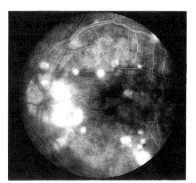

(b)

(c)

Figure 8.3 (*a*) Left fundus view of known case of sarcoidosis – note retinal oedema and pale subretinal granulomata. (*b*) and (*c*) Angiograms of (*a*) with early hyperfluoresence and subretinal lesions and later retinal and macular oedema, disc hyperfluorescence and staining of the upper temporal vein wall

pulmonary or mediastinal involvement, raised serum calcium, Kveim test, and radioisotope gallium scanning. Lymph node or conjunctival biopsy is confirmatory if these tissues are affected.

Treatment

Chronic macular oedema may lead to irreversible loss of central acuity and is a positive indication for treatment with steroids. The dosage is started at a high level – 60 or 80 mg per day reducing rapidly to a maintenance dose as low as possible.

Although vitreous inflammation may reduce vision this is not always a reason for treatment. If the disease process becomes inactive spontaneous clearing of the viteous gel will allow the vision to improve without intervention.

Topical steroid treatment for posterior segment disease is ineffective but may be required for concurrent anterior uveitis. Posterior sub-Tenon or orbital floor injections of depot steroids can be helpful.

Panretinal photocoagulation may be required for established proliferative neovascularization but it is advisable to try to reduce active inflammation by steroids first. In some cases neovascularization regresses after suppressing inflammation.

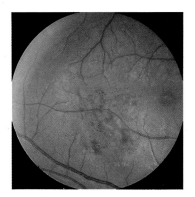

(a)

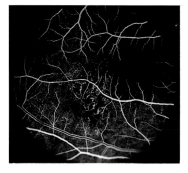

(b)

Behçet's disease

Behçet's disease is a chronic relapsing disease of unknown aetiology which affects young and middle-aged adults. It occurs world-wide but is found more commonly in the Mediterranean and Japan. It is a multisystem disorder mainly involving the skin, buccal mucous membrane and eyes but may also affect joints, gastrointestinal tract and the central nervous system. The disease has episodes of activity interposed with quiescent phases but the ultimate prognosis varies greatly from benign with little long-term deficit to severe central nervous system infarction and blindness.

Although the aetiology is unknown the disease is manifest as a vasculitis. A viral cause has been suggested but never proven; some patients have elevation of serum complement, circulating immune complexes and an association with HLA-B5 has been noted.

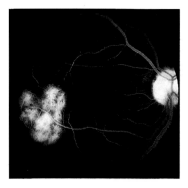

(c)

Figure 8.4 (*a*) Area of vascular disturbance in Behçets disease. (*b*) and (*c*) Angiogram of (*a*) showing retinal capillary dilatation, patchy closure and leakage in a territory based on the inferotemporal arteriole

Clinical features

The cardinal signs of Behçet's disease are aphthous ulcers of the buccal mucosa, genital or perineal skin ulceration and uveitis. The skin may also be affected by erythema nodosum or the joints by an inflammatory arthropathy. Some patients develop infarction in the central nervous system, particularly in the midbrain, and in these cases the prognosis for life can be poor.

The eyes are affected by anterior and posterior uveitis, retinal vasculitis or optic neuritis.

Anterior uveitis is usually bilateral and is often severe with patients presenting with a hypopyon. Signs in the posterior segment include vitreous cellular infiltration, white subretinal lesions and areas of retinal vasculitis and haemorrhages (Figure 8.4). When the optic nerve is affected by vasculitis there is a sudden profound fall in vision.

No reliable confirmatory test is available to prove the diagnosis, which therefore remains clinical. Needle pricks on the skin may lead to the development of small sterile skin abscesses and some patients have abnormal complement levels or circulating immune complexes.

Treatment

In addition to topical steroids and mydriatic agents to combat acute anterior uveitis systemic treatment is often necessary to control the condition. Both steroids and immunosuppressive agents are beneficial and are mandatory for optic neuritis or central nervous system disease. Initially prednisolone in high doses reducing over a few weeks should be used, but unresponsive cases may need chlorambucil, azathioprine or cyclosporin in addition. For the long term, a low-dose combination of prednisolone and an immunosuppressive drug will allow control of the disease, avoiding some of the side-effects of prolonged steroid administration. When immunosuppression is used regular blood counts to exclude bone-marrow depression and renal impairment should be performed.

Collagenoses

The collagen diseases are systemic conditions which affect many tissues of the body. The eyes are not commonly affected and ocular disease is rarely the main disability but in some patients symptoms can cause considerable discomfort and visual impairment can be severe.

Each of the collagen diseases tends to produce a particular ocular manifestation, e.g. rheumatoid arthritis causing nodular scleritis, but there is a large overlap in the affected tissues, thus almost any of the manifestations can be present with each of the conditions (Table 8.1).

Fundus abnormalities are not particularly common with the collagenoses but are well recognized in disseminated lupus erythematosus, polyarteritis nodosa and polymyositis. It should be borne in mind that systemic hypertension is common in these conditions and the retinal signs may be a

Table 8.1 Ocular manifestations of collagen diseases

	Rheumatoid arthritis	Disseminated lupus erythematosus	Polymyositis	Polyarteritis nodosa	Wegener's granulomatosis	Scleroderma
Dry eye	++	+	+	+	−	++
Keratitis	++	+	−	+	++	−
Scleritis	++	+	−	+	++	−
Uveitis	−	+	+	+	+	−
Retinal vasculitis	+	++	++	++	+	+
Optic neuritis	−	+	+	+	−	−

++ = well recognized association; + = uncommon association.

result of hypertensive retinopathy. However, in the absence of hypertension small vessel closure can be found in the retina with scattered retinal haemorrhages, cotton wool spots and arteriolar sheathing (Figure 8.5).

Detailed investigation and treatment of these systemic diseases is beyond the scope of this book and is best left in the hands of a specialist physician. Renal involvement is common but detailed radiological or haematological investigation varies according to the underlying diagnosis. A high erythrocyte sedimentation rate or plasma viscosity is universal. Circulating immune complexes have been found in SLE and polyarteritis nodosa.

Treatment

Treatment of the retinal vasculitis is part of the management of the generalized disease but sometimes requires specific attention. Rarely photocoagulation for proliferative retinopathy secondary to widespread retinal ischaemia may be required but the mainstay of treatment is systemic steroids, cytotoxic agents or a combination of both.

Syphilis

Syphilis is an uncommon cause of retinal vasculitis but investigation to exclude treponemal infection should always be performed in patients with vasculitis, particularly as active infection can be cured readily.

Clinical features

The fundus can be affected in both congenital and acquired infection by treponema pallidum.

Congenital syphilis

Congenital syphilitic chorioretinitis is a multifocal bilateral disorder producing a patchy pigmentary retinopathy – the salt and pepper fundus. On

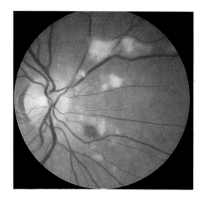

(a)

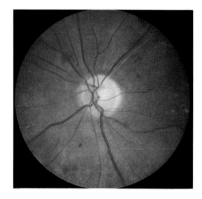

(b)

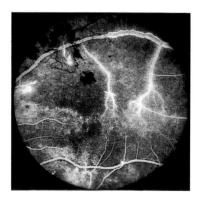

(c)

Figure 8.5 (*a*) Multiple cotton wool spots in polymyositis. (*b*) Longstanding arterial closure in SLE. (*c*) Angiogram of (*b*)

occasions the condition can mimic retinitis pigmentosa but the typical bone spicule pigmentation is not usually observed (Figure 8.6).

Postnatally the condition is inactive and does not require treatment. Refraction is necessary because of the common association of myopia, and special support, particularly for education, is required when vision is considerably reduced.

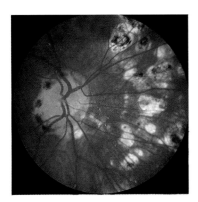

Figure 8.6 Multifocal chorioretinal scars from congenital syphilis

Acquired syphilis

Acquired syphilis affects the retina during the secondary stage, usually 4–6 weeks after initial infection.

Some degree of uveitis and vitreous haze is usually present which can obscure a detailed view of the retina. Direct retinal involvement produces white retinal infiltrative lesions with variable degrees of vasculitis (Figure 8.7).

Fluorescein angiography shows the retinitis to be hypofluorescent followed by staining but there is widespread dye leakage from the surrounding capillary bed (Figure 8.7).

Serological tests for syphilis should not rely on the Wassermann reaction alone as false positives occur; Venereal Disease Research Laboratory tests and fluorescent treponemal antibody tests should also be performed. Yaws yields genuine positive reactions to treponemal serological tests and patients coming from areas where yaws is endemic can present difficulties in diagnosis.

Treatment for active syphilis is a 3-week course of injections of intramuscular benzyl penicillin.

Initial treatment with a week of intravenous penicillin has also been advocated.

Optic atrophy is a further manifestation of syphilis. This occurs in the tertiary stage of the disease which can be many years after primary infection. Optic atrophy results from small vessel occlusion and endarteritis obliterans.

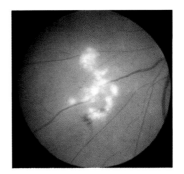

(*a*)

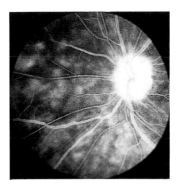

(*b*)

Figure 8.7 (*a*) Acute retinal infiltration during secondary syphilis. (*b*) Angiogram of (*a*) showing widespread retinal oedema and dye leakage

Acquired immune deficiency syndrome (AIDS)

AIDS is caused by a retrovirus, human immunodeficiency virus (HIV), of which there are two subtypes. Type 1 is currently world-wide and is reponsible for the increasing numbers of patients found to be suffering from AIDS. The United States of America and central Africa are particularly affected but infection is rapidly involving most countries of the world.

The virus affects subsets of the T lymphocytes leading to deficiency of helper cells. B lymphocytes are also affected to some degree as circulating antibody responses to secondary infection are usually non-specific and inappropriate.

The virus is shed in body fluids. Semen, saliva and tears have all been shown to contain virus but transmission is mainly by sexual contact, particularly by homosexual practices. An increasing number of women are now becoming affected, usually from bisexual partners, but patients receiving transfusions of blood or blood products and intravenous drug abusers are also at risk of contracting the disease. No known case of cross-infection from tears has been recorded.

Clinical features

The primary infection results in a mild systemic disease with malaise and lymphadenopathy. Thereafter there is a latent phase with no obvious clinical manifestations but affected patients are seropositive for HIV. After the latent phase, which may last several years, the patient develops the full syndrome with malaise, weight loss, lymphadenopathy and secondary opportunistic infections from immune deficiency. It is not known what proportion of patients who are seropositive later develop the full syndrome but the number is high and probably well over 50%.

Systemic secondary infections usually affect the lungs, central nervous system and the gastrointestinal tract. *Pneumocystis carinii* pneumonia, meningitis from *Cryptococcus neoformans*, encephalitis from *Toxoplasma gondii* and intestinal cytomegalovirus or candida infection are common.

Ophthalmic involvement is mainly by Kaposi's sarcoma of the conjunctiva or orbit and by retinopathy.

Typically the retinopathy is manifest by cotton wool spots from scattered microinfarcts in the retina together with retinal haemorrhages and intraretinal microvascular abnormalities. These lesions may represent direct infection or be the result of circulating immune complexes (Figure 8.8).

Vision is minimally affected initially but frequently the retinopathy may be much more fulminant as a result of cytomegalovirus infection. In such cases the retinopathy can be observed to

start as white patches in the peripheral retina which gradually expand as the virus spreads to infect neighbouring cells. There is complete retinal destruction in the affected areas with loss of function. The process, if left untreated, progresses inexorably to destroy wide areas of the retina and causes blindness. Cytomegalovirus retinopathy is usually found towards the terminal stages of AIDS infection and patients do not often survive for more than 6 months.

Serological testing for HIV infection is by detecting antibodies against both virus capsule and core antigens. The capsule antibody remains positive once seroconversion has occurred after primary infection. Core antibodies revert to negative but become positive again once the syndrome becomes active later in the disease.

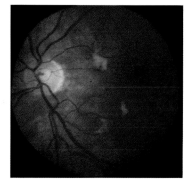

(a)

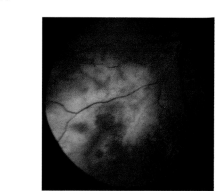

(b)

Figure 8.8 (*a*) Microinfarcts from AIDS infection. (*b*) Cytomegalo-virus retinitis. (Reproduced by courtesy of Mr R. J. Marsh.)

Treatment

Treatment for the systemic condition is by azidothymidine (AZT) which prolongs life but is only palliative. Cytomegalovirus retinopathy has been shown to become inactive after using dihydroxypropoxymethyl guanine (DHPG) but once the treatment is discontinued the retinopathy reactivates. Repeated courses are therefore required. Patients who develop bone marrow suppression from systemic drug treatment can be treated by repeated intravitreous injections but multiple doses are needed.

Acute retinal necrosis

This rare but very grave ocular disorder affects middle-aged adults and is usually bilateral. Although the aetiology is not fully known some patients have been described with rising titres of antibodies against herpes simplex virus and in others possible zoster infection has been implicated.

Clinical features

The presenting feature of acute retinal necrosis is a severe uveitis. This can be so marked that a hypopyon is present and the retinal signs are either overlooked or not visible through the accompanying dense vitreous infiltration with inflammatory cells.

Vision in an affected eye is severely reduced. The retinal signs usually begin in the periphery near the equator and appear as extensive dense white, well-demarcated areas of necrotic retina. Patchy ischaemic retinal haemorrhages may also be seen. The larger retinal vessels are usually visible in stark relief against the white retinal background (Figure 8.9).

The areas of necrosis tend to increase and the peripheral retina becomes necrotic with the formation of large tears and secondary retinal detachment.

Treatment

Systemic and topical steroids are used to suppress the concurrent uveitis but they are not effective against the retinal necrosis and do not appear to prevent the high incidence of retinal detachment. Oral acyelovir should be tried in those patients in whom herpes simplex is suspected. Scleral buckling procedures and vitrectomy may result in retinal reapposition in some cases but visual function is usually poor as a result of marked optic atrophy.

Pars planitis (intermediate uveitis)

Pars planitis is a specific form of uveitis of the posterior segment which may also be accompanied by retinal vasculitis. The condition may be unilateral but in the majority of cases is bilateral. Affected patients are usually young adults and it is not uncommonly found in teenagers. The aetiology is unknown.

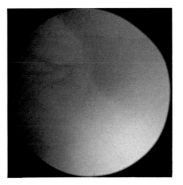

(a)

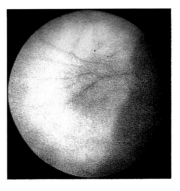

(b)

Figure 8.9 (a) Acute retinal necrosis. (b) Red free photograph of (a)

Clinical features

The hallmarks of the condition are vitreous cellular infiltration, together with white cellular masses in the inferior peripheral vitreous (snowballs) and a grey–white exudate overlying the pars plana (snow-banking). Snow-banking is typically found inferiorly but in severe cases extends round over the temporal and nasal pars plana (Figure 8.10). Accompanying signs which may be present are of a variably severe anterior uveitis, macular oedema (Figure 8.11) and peripheral vasculitis with periphlebeal sheathing, small retinal haemorrhages and vessel closure. In severe cases retinal exudation and peripheral neovascularization may occur.

The clinical course of the disease is relatively benign in many cases with vision mildly reduced by anterior uveitis and vitreous debris. In some patients vision is seriously affected by dense vitreous opacity and by chronic macular oedema leading to cystoid spaces in the neuroretina. Rarely, severe visual loss occurs from peripheral neovascularization and vitreous haemorrhage.

Fluorescein angiography is not usually helpful in the diagnosis of pars planitis although, if performed, intense dye leakage can be observed from the retinal periphery. Angiography can be useful in identifying and monitoring the presence and severity of capillary leakage at the macula and the response to treatment.

Treatment

Treatment of pars planitis can sometimes be difficult to judge. The course of the disease is protracted over many years and it is important that the treatment does not leave the patient more debilitated than the disease process itself.

Anterior uveitis should be controlled by topical medication with mydriatics and steroids. This is important to prevent the long-term complications of anterior uveitis such as posterior synechiae and also to maintain the view of the posterior segment where the more serious aspects of the disease occur. However, topical steroids do not ameliorate posterior segment disease.

Vitreous cellular debris does not usually require systemic treatment unless vision is seriously affected but in these circumstances macular oedema is often present at the same time. Subconjunctival, sub-Tenon's capsule or orbital floor injections of depot steroid preparations can be tried as a temporary measure to reduce inflammation but are not usually a long-term solution for this protracted disease.

Once visual acuity is reduced significantly from chronic macular oedema, treatment by systemic steroids should be started. Initially moderately high doses are used and then reduced after 2 or 3 weeks. Attempts should be made every few

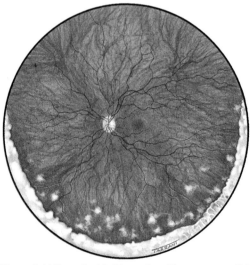

Figure 8.10 Pars planitis (Reproduced by courtesy of Mr T. Tarrant)

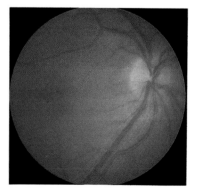

Figure 8.11 Cystoid macular oedema secondary to pars planitis

months to wean off steroids completely but sometimes macular oedema recurs requiring prolonged steroid treatment which is unfortunate in these young patients. If steroid dosage has to be maintained at a high level, immunosuppressive agents such as azathioprine or chlorambucil can be tried instead or in addition.

When severe peripheral retinal vasculitis is present leading to extensive exudate deposition or neovascularization additional treatment may be required. Photocoagulation is not usually helpful as the lesions are too peripheral for three-mirror examination, therefore cryotherapy to the pre-equatorial retina may be the treatment of choice.

In the long term cataracts are a frequent complication both from the disease and from steroid treatment. When they occur they can be managed by extracapsular surgery in a standard way.

Preretinal gliosis affecting the macula is a common complication of longstanding pars planitis and care must be taken not to confuse this with persistent macular oedema, thereby prolonging steroid usage unnecessarily. Fluorescein angiography may be helpful in differentiating cellophane from cystoid maculopathy.

Further reading

BOECK, J. (1956) Ocular changes in periarteritis nodosa. *American Journal of Ophthalmology*, **42**, 567–576

DUANE, T. D. Ocular manifestations of connective tissue disorders. In *Clinical Ophthalmology*, Vol. V, Chapter 26, Harper and Row, New York

DUANE, T. D. Retinal vasculitis. In *Clinical Ophthalmology*, Vol. IV, Chapter 47, Harper and Row, New York

FFYTCHE, T. J. (1977) Retinal vasculitis. *Transactions of the Ophthalmological Society of the UK*, **97**, 457–461

FREEMAN, W. R., THOMAS, E. L., RAO, N. A. and PEPOSE, J. S. (1986) Demonstration of herpes group virus in acute retinal necrosis syndrome. *American Journal of Ophthalmology*, **102**, 701–709

GOLD, D. H., MORRIS, D. A. and HENKIND, P. (1972) Ocular findings in systemic lupus erythematosus. *British Journal of Ophthalmology*, **56**, 800–804

GRAHAM, E. M., STANFORD, M. R., SHILLING, J. S. and SANDERS, M. D. (1987) Neovascularisation associated with posterior uveitis. *British Journal of Ophthalmology*, **71**, 826–833

GRAHAM, E. M., STANFORD, M. R., SANDERS, M. D., KASP, E. and DUMONDE, D. C. (1989) A point prevalence study of 150 patients with idiopathic retinal vasculitis I and II. *British Journal of Ophthalmology*, **73**, 714–730

HUMPHREY, R. C., WEBER, J. N. and MARSH, R. J. (1987) Ophthalmic findings in a group of ambulatory patients infected by human immunodeficiency virus (HIV). *British Journal of Ophthalmology*, **71**, 565–569

OBENAUF, C. D., SHAW, H. E., SYDNOR, C. F. and KLINTWORTH, G. K. (1978) Sarcoidosis and its ocular manifestations. *American Journal of Ophthalmology*, **86**, 648–655

ORELLANA, J., TEICH, S. A., WINTERKORN, J. S., MATHUR-WAGH, U., HANDWERGER, S. and SCHLAMM, H. (1988) Treatment of cytomegalovirus retinitis with gancyclovir. *British Journal of Ophthalmology*, **72**, 525–529

PEDERSON, J. E., KENYON, K. R., GREEN, W. R. and MAUMENEE, A. E. (1978) Pathology of pars planitis. *American Journal of Ophthalmology*, **86**, 762–774

RAHI, A. H. S. and GARNER, A. (1976) *Immunopathology of the Eye*, Blackwell Scientific Publications, Oxford

SPALTON, D. J. and SANDERS, M. D. (1981) Fundus changes in histologically confirmed sarcoidosis. *British Journal of Ophthalmology*, **65**, 348–358

SPENCER, W. H. (1985) Inflammatory diseases and conditions. In *Ophthalmic Pathology*, Vol. II, Chapter 8, W. B. Saunders, Philadelphia

STANFORD, M. R., GRAHAM, E., KASP, E. and SANDERS, M. D. (1988) A longitudinal study of clinical and immunological findings in 52 patients with relapsing retinal vasculitis. *British Journal of Ophthalmology*, **72**, 442–447

WAKEFIELD, D., EASTER, J., BREIT, S. N., CLARK, P. and PENNY, R. (1985) α antitrypsin serum levels and phenotypes in patients with retinal vasculitis. *British Journal of Ophthalmology*, **69**, 497–499

YOUNG, N. J. A. and BIRD, A. C. (1978) Bilateral acute retinal necrosis. *British Journal of Ophthalmology*, **62**, 581–590

9

Retinal disease with blood disorders

Disorders of red blood cells

Anaemia

Retinal vascular disturbance resulting from anaemia is not commonly encountered in routine ophthalmic practice in Western countries. If anaemia becomes severe and circulating haemoglobin is reduced to less than half-normal levels, changes in the fundus may develop.

Anaemia may be a result of increased blood loss (hypochromic or iron deficiency), reduced red cell production (vitamin B12 deficiency or aplastic) or of increased haemolysis. With the exception of the haemoglobinopathies such as sickle cell disease (see p. 45) the ophthalmoscopic appearances are not characteristic of the type of anaemia, and diagnosis depends on analysis of the blood film.

Clinical features

The fundus appearance resulting from anaemia is one of scattered retinal haemorrhages, either flame shaped in the nerve fibre layer or blot in the deeper layers (Figure 9.1). Unless a haemorrhage occurs at the macula vision is usually unaffected but occasionally haemorrhages may be more extensive and rupture through into the subhyaloid space. Cotton wool spots and optic disc swelling have been noted in severe anaemia and are presumed to result from localized ischaemia.

In cases of acute blood loss patients may develop severe visual disturbance from infarction of the visual pathways. Normally this occurs at the

optic disc head, giving rise to arcuate, quadrantic or hemispheral field defects, or in the occipital cortex leading to hemianopia.

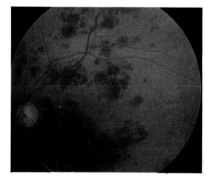

(a)

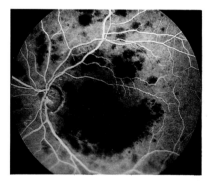

(b)

Figure 9.1 (a) Diffuse retinal haemorrhages associated with severe anaemia (haemoglobin concentration 5.2 g 100 ml^{-1} (0.81 mmol l^{-1})). (b) Angiogram of (a). Multiple areas of masking with closure of macular capillary bed

Treatment

Treatment of the anaemia results in reversal of the retinal signs and specific ocular treatment is not required. Visual prognosis is good unless severe retinal or optic nerve infarction has occurred. In cases of vitamin B12 deficiency there may be an accompanying optic neuropathy as well as the anaemia which requires long-term hydroxycobalamin injections.

Polycythaemia

Polycythaemia rubra vera is a proliferative condition affecting the bone marrow causing an increase in the number of circulating red blood cells. A secondary form of polycythaemia follows raised blood carbon dioxide from chronic lung disease and emphysema. The diagnosis is established by finding a high haematocrit from the increased red cell mass.

Clinical features

Qualitatively the retinal changes caused by primary or secondary polycythaemia are similar and result from the mechanical rheological problems from the increased circulating red cell mass. There is an increase in retinal venous tortuosity and darkening of the blood column. The picture may progress to that of central retinal vein occlusion with optic disc swelling and scattered retinal haemorrhages. Unfortunately the condition can be bilateral and can result in severe visual loss.

Treatment of polycythaemia rubra vera by venesection decreases the venous tortuosity and provided venous occlusion has not taken place the outlook for vision is good. Advice from a physician is required for management of the polycythaemia whether primary or secondary. Once venous occlusion has taken place management of the retina is the same as for other cases of central vein occlusion (see Chapter 4).

Disorders of white blood cells

Leukaemia

Leukaemia may be acute or chronic and affect either the myelocytic, lymphocytic or monocytic series of blood cells. They are all characterized by neoplastic proliferation of the affected group of white cells with a greatly increased count in the circulating peripheral blood.

Clinical features

Ocular signs are more common in acute than chronic disease but the fundus picture is not diagnostic for any particular type of leukaemia. As well as fundus involvement the conjunctiva is frequently infiltrated, which can be useful for diagnostic biopsy (Figure 9.2).

The choroid and the retina may both be affected by leukaemic infiltration. When choroidal invasion occurs there is a patchy pallor of the background appearance of the fundus which can be easily overlooked. Retinal signs are much easier to observe and consist of vessel sheathing venous dilatation, white infiltrative masses within the neuroretina and multiple retinal haemorrhages (Figure 9.3). Sometimes the haemorrhages have white centres similar to Roth's spots. Multifocal areas of infarction of the neuroretina with cotton wool spots are common and may severely reduce vision. Direct infiltration of the optic nerve head by leukaemic deposits are a serious manifestation with a poor visual outlook.

Treatment

The prognosis for survival with leukaemia has greatly improved during the past two decades and management with chemotherapy is best left in the hands of the specialist. Resolution of the ocular

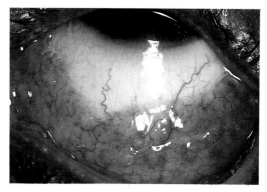

Figure 9.2 Leukaemia infiltration of the conjunctiva

signs follows improvement of the underlying leukaemia and specific ocular treatment is usually not required. In those cases where visual loss is more profound or imminent, localized radiotherapy to reduce retinal infiltration should be considered.

In rare cases severe retinal ischaemia leads to vasoproliferative retinopathy, which needs laser panretinal photocoagulation.

Reticulum cell sarcoma

Reticulum cell sarcoma presents rarely to the ophthalmologist. However, the central nervous system and eye may be exclusively affected and diagnosis can be difficult.

Clinical features

Affected patients usually present with uveitis but later the vitreous may become completely opaque with white cells and the choroid infiltrated by multiple deposits. Secondary retinal detachment may follow.

Treatment

Diagnostic vitrectomy and histology of the excised vitreous reveals the nature of the disease enabling chemotherapy or radiotherapy to be instigated.

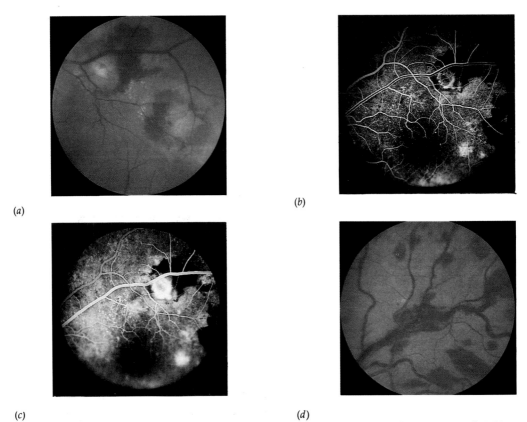

(a)

(b)

(c)

(d)

Figure 9.3 (*a*) Retinal infiltration and haemorrhage in acute lymphocytic leukaemia. (*b*) Angiogram of (*a*). Note early fluorescence (*b*) and intense late staining (*c*) of infiltrate. (*d*) Lymphocytic lymphoma. Note typical pale centred haemorrhage

Dysproteinaemias

Waldenström's macroglobulinaemia and multiple myeloma are diseases in which there is an increase in circulating gamma globulins. In the former there is an increase in IgM and in the latter an abnormal IgG is produced.

The effect of the increase in protein is to greatly increase the blood viscosity with sludging of the retinal circulation.

Clinical features

Initially there is an increase in venous tortuosity which may be extreme. Exudates or haemorrhages may be seen and frank venous occlusion in the retina is common (Figure 9.4).

Treatment

Early retinal signs will reverse if the condition is treated by plasmapheresis. Vein occlusions require management, as outlined in Chapter 4, to prevent the complications of new vessel formation and rubeotic glaucoma.

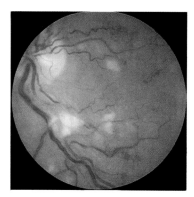

(a)

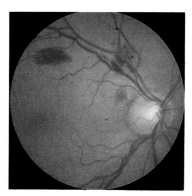

(b)

Figure 9.4 (*a*) Fundus appearance in a case of Waldenström's macroglobulinaemia. (*b*) Fundus appearance in a case of multiple myeloma

Further reading

ACKERMAN, A. L. (1962) Ocular manifestations of Waldenström's macroglobulinaemia and its treatment. *Archives of Ophthalmology*, **67**, 701–707

AISEN, M. L., BACON, B. R., GOODMAN, A. M. and CHESTER, E. M. (1983) Retinal abnormalities associated with anaemia. *Archives of Ophthalmology*, **101**, 1049–1052

ALLAN, R. A. and STRAATSMA, B. R. (1961) Ocular involvement in leukaemia and allied disorders. *Archives of Ophthalmology*, **66**, 490–508

DUANE, T. D. Retinopathy of blood dyscrasias. In *Clinical Ophthalmology*, Vol. III, Chapter 18, Harper and Row, New York

DUANE, T. D. Haematological disorders. In *Clinical Ophthalmology*, Vol. V, Chapter 23, Harper and Row, New York

MERIN, S. and FREUND, M. (1968) Retinopathy in severe anaemia. *American Journal of Ophthalmology*, **66**, 1102–1106

SIEGEL, M. J., DALTON, J., FRIEDMAN, A. H., STRAUCHEN, J. and WATSON, C. (1989) Ten year experience with primary ocular reticulum cell sarcoma. *British Journal of Ophthalmology*, **73**, 342–346

SPENCER, W. H. (1985) Systemic diseases with retinal involvement. In *Ophthalmic Pathology*, Vol. II, Chapter 8, W. B. Saunders, Philadelphia

10

Miscellaneous retinal vascular conditions

Cystoid macular oedema

Cystoid macular oedema is not a diagnosis *per se* but occurs secondary to disease processes affecting the blood–retinal barrier. Breakdown of either the inner or outer blood–retinal barrier can result in fluid accumulation in the plexiform layers of the parafoveal neuroretina. Chronic oedema leads to the development of cystic spaces, which are most easily viewed biomicroscopically at the slit lamp, and produces a characteristic picture on fluorescein angiography. In the early stages of the dye transit the parafoveal capillaries are dilated and then gradually leak. The cystoid spaces around the fovea fill with dye to produce a typical petaloid pattern.

Many retinal disorders induce cystoid macular oedema but the pathogenesis can be broadly classified into: (a) postoperative, (b) toxic, (c) dystrophic, (d) secondary to retinal vascular disease, (e) secondary to subretinal fluid.

Postoperative cystoid macular oedema

Intracapsular cataract extraction is followed for a few weeks after surgery by cystoid oedema in 50% of cases when subjected to fluorescein angiography (Figure 10.1). Ophthalmoscopically oedema is not always easily visible and it does not appear to have significant bearing on visual acuity. In nearly all cases the oedema resolves over a period of months with no lasting sequelae. The incidence of cystoid oedema with extracapsular cataract extraction is less than 5%.

In cases of cataract extraction complicated by vitreous incarceration into the incision there is a high incidence of persistent cystoid oedema which slowly but increasingly impairs visual acuity. This condition, called the vitreous wick syndrome, may result from vitreous traction on the posterior retina by vitreous strands in the wound. In some cases with posterior vitreous detachment no such strands can be demonstrated and it is presumed that low-grade iritis from pupillary distortion causes the macular oedema. The treatment of the syndrome is by vitrectomy to clear the vitreous from the anterior segment, iris and anterior vitreous cavity. Postoperatively the oedema resolves but surgery is best performed before visual acuity is seriously reduced because recovery is poor in some cases. Acetazolamide can be tried before surgery but the result is usually disappointing.

Other forms of intraocular surgery have also been shown to cause cystoid macular oedema, particularly glaucoma surgery and keratoplasty. Ocular hypotony may have a role in the cause of macular oedema in such cases because persistently soft eyes frequently develop cystoid changes at the macula and optic disc swelling.

Toxic cystoid macular oedema

Topical adrenaline or high doses of oral nicotinamide have been shown to cause cystoid macular oedema. The condition resolves when the drug is discontinued.

In cases of oedema following topical adrenaline the problem occurs only in certain patients and

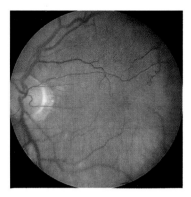

(a)

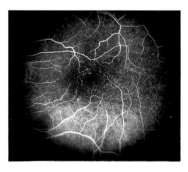

(b)

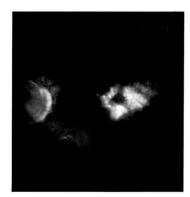

(c)

Figure 10.1 (a) Cystoid macular oedema following intracapsular cataract extraction. (b) and (c) Angiograms of (a). Vascular changes (b) and oedema (c) much easier seen on angiography

only after intracapsular cataract surgery. The reaction appears to be an idiosyncracy but aphakic patients starting adrenaline drops for glaucoma should be observed carefully. If oedema does not develop after a few weeks it is unlikely to do so even after prolonged usage.

Dystrophic cystoid macular oedema

Cystoid macular oedema may occur as a result of inherited fundus dystrophies. On rare occasions it can be found as an isolated dominantly inherited condition but may also be seen in cases of retinitis pigmentosa or photoreceptor dystrophies.

Widespread retinal capillary leakage can be observed in some cases of retinitis pigmentosa and on occasions is severe enough to produce cystoid macular spaces. It is not known whether this is an effect of a defective pigment epithelium or is a result of retinal capillary endothelial damage. The incidence is higher in cases with vitreous inflammatory cells and the oedema may, therefore, be a result of low-grade inflammation.

Retinitis pigmentosa patients developing cystoid oedema lose central acuity which can be very disabling in view of the already restricted peripheral vision. Oral steroids or acetazolamide may be tried in an attempt to reduce oedema. Grid photocoagulation has been used by some with reported morphological improvement.

Cystoid macular oedema secondary to retinal vascular disease

Chronic retinal capillary leakage frequently follows both retinal vein obstruction and inflammatory vessel disease. In mild central vein occlusion, once the acute disturbance has resolved, the only evidence of vascular damage in some cases is the presence of persistent macular oedema. Ultimately this tends to resolve over a period of years leaving underlying pigment epithelial mottling but central vision remains poor. The treatment of retinal vein obstruction has been described already (see Chapter 4).

Pars planitis, sarcoidosis, toxoplasmosis and other forms of retinal vasculitis frequently induce macular oedema which may develop a cystoid pattern if it becomes prolonged. Treatment depends on the underlying cause (see Chapter 8).

Cystoid macular oedema secondary to subretinal fluid

Chronic accumulation of fluid in the subretinal space at the macula often leads to the formation of cystoid spaces at the fovea. The fluid may be the result of leakage through the retinal pigment epithelium (disciform degeneration, choroidal tumours) or from subretinal fluid associated with rhegmatogenous retinal detachment (Figure 10.2).

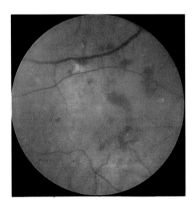

(a)

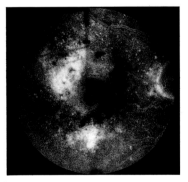

(b)

Figure 10.2 (*a*) Cystoid macular oedema following subretinal fluid secondary to ageing disciform degeneration. (*b*) Angiogram of (*a*) showing diffuse intraretinal leakage at the fovea

In most instances the presence of cystoid oedema does not produce symptoms as the major cause of visual loss is the primary disease. However, if the underlying condition is successfully treated, cystoid oedema may limit the recovery of visual acuity. It should be borne in mind that surgery for rhegmatogenous retinal detachment may also produce cystoid macular oedema as a postoperative complication.

Some patients with preretinal traction membranes develop cystoid macular oedema but this occurs in those cases with severe traction and frequently there is shallow subretinal fluid present (Figure 10.3).

Radiation retinopathy

A wide variety of ocular and orbital conditions require treatment by radiotherapy as a necessary part of their management. The most commonly encountered disorders requiring such treatment are dysthyroid eye disease and malignancies affecting the orbit, choroid and paranasal sinuses.

Radiotherapy is administered either by external beam or by radioactive plaques containing cobalt or ruthenium sutured to the sclera. The retinopathy is similar regardless of the type of radiotherapy employed. Although there is a wide personal variation in susceptibility it is suggested 3000 rads (30 Gy) or more is likely to induce retinopathy. The capillary endothelial cells become damaged and the small arterioles hyalinized. The blood–retinal barrier is defective with oedema and exudate deposition and, if capillary closure is extensive, retinal hypoxia and vascular proliferation follow.

The retinopathy becomes manifest after an interval of months or years following the course of radiotherapy. Clinically the appearance is similar to that of diabetic retinopathy with focal areas of microvascular changes, capillary closure and leakage (Figures 10.4 and 10.5).

Management is along the lines of other disorders producing exudation or ischaemia. Macular oedema may respond to focal laser treatment and proliferative retinopathy to panretinal photocoagulation. Unfortunately in some patients the retinopathy is progressive with a poor visual outlook and there is a high incidence of neovascular glaucoma in severe cases.

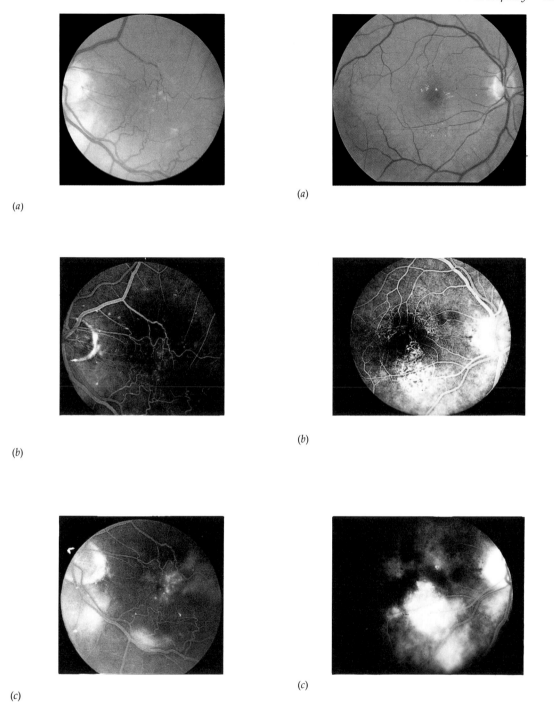

(*a*)

(*b*)

(*c*)

(*a*)

(*b*)

(*c*)

Figure 10.3 (*a*) Preretinal traction membrane causing vascular distortion and oedema. (*b*) and (*c*) Angiograms of (*a*)

Figure 10.4 (*a*) Mild radiation retinopathy following therapy for orbital meningioma 20 years previously. (*b*) and (*c*) Angiograms of (*a*) showing widespread capillary dilatation and leakage

Radioactive plaques sutured to the sclera to treat melanoma or retinoblastoma close to the posterior pole of the eye may produce an acute optic disc swelling and subsequent optic atrophy.

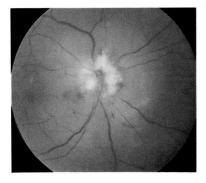

(a)

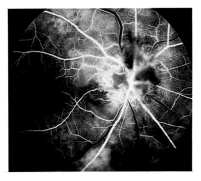

(b)

Figure 10.5 (*a*) Severe optic disc swelling 2 years after radiation for choroidal metastasis. (*b*) Angiogram of (*a*) showing capillary leakage and areas of closure of the peripapillary plexus

Purtscher's retinopathy

Severe trauma to the body as experienced in road traffic accidents or falls from heights may be followed by a retinopathy, even in the absence of direct ocular trauma. The exact mechanism producing the retinal vascular changes is unknown but complex multiple factors are probably present leading to focal areas of retinal infarction. Fractures of long bones can produce fat emboli and such lesions have been found in the retinal circulation. Crush injuries to the chest cause sudden severe increases in venous pressure resulting in valsalva haemorrhages. Also, severe trauma may induce intravascular coagulopathy and thereby increase retinal infarction.

Ophthalmoscopically, the retinopathy tends to be most obvious around the optic disc and posterior pole. White areas in the nerve fibre layer from presumed arteriolar obstruction surround the disc. Patchy haemorrhages are seen, some of which are deep, resembling those of infarction, and some superficial under the internal limiting lamina, similar to those seen after valsalva (Figure 10.6). Unlike valsalva haemorrhages, which clear without serious visual complications, Purtscher's retinopathy causes reduced vision as a result of infarction and optic atrophy.

A similar fundoscopic picture is sometimes seen in patients with acute pancreatitis.

Leber's optic atrophy

This inherited disorder causes acute loss of vision in one eye followed a few days, weeks or months later by a similar episode in the fellow eye.

The pattern of inheritance is unusual. There is a large preponderance of affected males and succeeding generations may be affected, suggesting X-linked inheritance, but:

1. Males do not transmit the disease onwards.
2. Females transmit the disease to 50% of sons but only 10% of daughters.
3. All the daughters of an affected female seem to be carriers.

The disease may be transmitted by cytoplasmic inheritance or by an infective agent such as a slow virus.

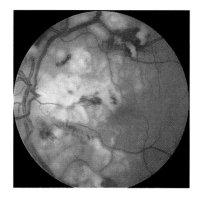

(a)

Optic nerve involvement occurs in the second or third decade of life with loss of central vision developing over a few days. The optic disc appears slightly swollen and the peripapillary retinal capillaries are mildly dilated and tortuous. There may be abnormal capillary hyperfluorescence during angiography, but in some cases there is no leakage in spite of clinically dilated capillaries (Figure 10.7). The fellow eye usually becomes affected sooner or later which can be a pointer in establishing the diagnosis.

Recovery of central vision is usually poor but the peripheral fields remain full. Courses of systemic steroids and hydroxycobalamin have been tried but have not proven helpful.

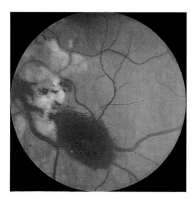

(b)

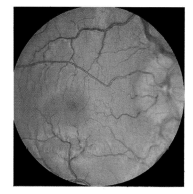

(a)

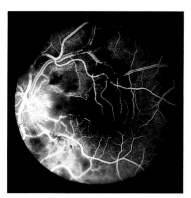

(c)

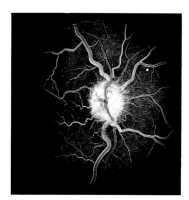

(b)

Figure 10.6 (a) Purtscher's retinopathy with multiple cotton wool spots and retinal haemorrhages. (b) Purtscher's retinopathy with superficial valsalva haemorrhage under the internal limiting lamina. (c) Angiogram of (a) showing capillary closure

Figure 10.7 (a) Leber's optic atrophy in a 16-year-old boy. (b) Angiography shows capillary leakage, which is absent in some cases

Leber's stellate maculopathy

Leber's stellate maculopathy is an unusual benign condition affecting healthy adults.

Vision is mildly affected by the formation of a macular star of exudate secondary to mild optic disc swelling (Figure 10.8). No underlying neurological abnormality of the optic nerve is found but fluorescein angiography demonstrates mild disc leakage. The exudate in the outer plexiform layer resembles the macular star seen in other forms of optic disc swelling such as that seen in papilloedema secondary to raised intracranial pressure.

The disease is self-limiting and the exudate clears over several months with good visual recovery.

Congenital hypertrophy of the retinal pigment epithelium

Small areas of hypertrophied, hyperpigmented patches of the retinal pigment epithelium are not uncommon. Usually there is no associated neuroretinal defect but sometimes larger lesions have coarsening or absence of the overlying retinal capillaries (Figure 10.9). The changes appear to be of no clinical significance.

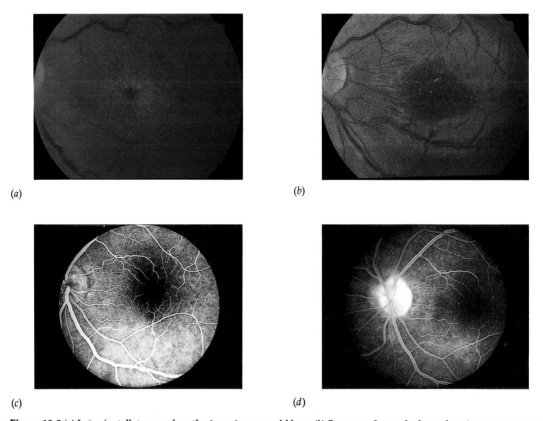

(a)   (b)

(c)   (d)

Figure 10.8 (*a*) Leber's stellate maculopathy in a nine year old boy. (*b*) Same eye 3 months later showing spontaneous resolution (Courtesy of Mr G. Sturrock). (*c*) and (*d*) Angiogram of a 23-year-old man with stellate maculopathy showing normal retinal capillaries but disc hypercornia

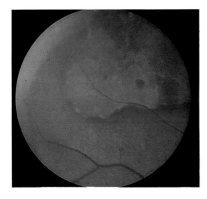

(a)

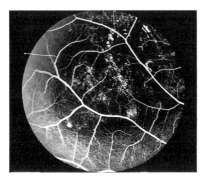

(b)

Figure 10.9 (*a*) Congenital hypertrophy of the retinal pigment epithelium. (*b*) Angiogram of (*a*) showing ·coarsening of the retinal capillary network

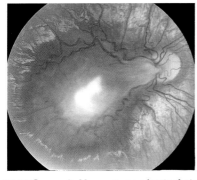

Figure 10.10 Congenital hamartoma of retinal pigment epithelium with retinal involvement

Congenital hyperplasia (hamartoma) of the retinal pigment epithelium

This very rare hamartomatous defect usually presents in childhood or early adult life. It consists of a mass of thickened hyperplastic pigment epithelium with overlying retinal fibrosis and vascular dilatation and tortuosity. The blood–retinal barrier is usually preserved with no marked exudation of the retina. The lesions may occur close to the optic disc or in the retinal periphery (Figure 10.10).

Vision is poor where the macula is involved but no treatment is available.

Further reading

BAGAN, S. M. and HOLLENHORST, R. W. (1979) Radiation retinopathy after irradiation of intracranial lesions. *American Journal of Ophthalmology*, **88**, 694–697

BECKINGSALE, A. B. and ROSENTHAL, A. R. (1983) Early fundus fluorescein angiographic findings and sequelae in traumatic retinopathy. *British Journal of Ophthalmology*, **67**, 119–123

BROWN, G. C., SHIELDS, J. A., SANBORN, G., AUGSBURGER, J. J., SAVINO, P. J. and SCHATZ, N. J. (1982) Radiation retinopathy. *Ophthalmology*, **89**, 1494–1501

CAROLL, D. M. and FRANKLIN, R. M. (1982) Leber's idiopathic stellate retinopathy. *American Journal of Ophthalmology*, **93**, 96–101

CHEE, P. H. Y. (1968) Radiation retinopathy. *American Journal of Ophthalmology*, **66**, 860–865

CLEARY, P. E., GREGOR, Z. and BIRD, A. C. (1976) Retinal vascular changes in congenital hypertrophy of the retinal pigment epithelium. *British Journal of Ophthalmology*, **60**, 499–503

COX, S. N., HAY, E. and BIRD, A. C. (1988) Treatment of chronic macular oedema with acetazolamide. *Archives of Ophthalmology*, **106**, 1190–1195

DREYER, R. F., HOPEN, G., GASS, J. D. M. and SMITH, J. L. (1984) Leber's idiopathic stellate neuroretinitis. *Archives of Ophthalmology*, **102**, 1140–1145

DUANE, T. D. Leber's stellate maculopathy. In *Clinical Ophthalmology*, Vol. III, Chapter 23, Harper and Row, New York

DUANE, T. D. Leber's disease. In *Clinical Ophthalmology*, Vol. 2, Chapter 5, Harper and Row, New York

FFYTCH, T. J. (1972) Cystoid maculopathy in retinitis pigmentosa. *Transactions of the Ophthalmological Society of the UK*, **92**, 265–283

FINE, B. S. and BRUCKER, A. J. (1981) Macular oedema and cystoid macular oedema. *American Journal of Ophthalmology*, **92**, 466–481

FRANÇOIS, J., VERRIEST, G. and DE LAEY, J. J. (1969) Leber's idiopathic stellate retinopathy. *American Journal of Ophthalmology*, **68**, 340–345

GASS, J. D. M. (1973) Nicotinic acid maculopathy. *American Journal of Ophthalmology*, **76**, 500–510

GASS, J. D. M. (1987) *Stereoscopic Atlases of Macular Diseases*, 3rd edn., C. V. Mosby, New York

HITCHINGS, R. A. (1977) Aphakic macular oedema: a two year follow up study. *British Journal of Ophthalmology*, **61**, 628–630

HITCHINGS, R. A. and CHISHOLM, I. H. (1975) Incidence of aphakic macular oedema. *British Journal of Ophthalmology*, **59**, 444–450

INKELES, D. M. and WALSH, J. M. (1975) Retinal fat emboli as a sequela to acute pancreatitis. *American Journal of Ophthalmology*, **80**, 935–938

KELLEY, J. S. (1974) Purtscher's retinopathy related to chest compression by safety belts. *American Journal of Ophthalmology*, **74**, 278–283

KINCAID, M. C., GREEN, W. R., KNOX, D. L. and MOHLER, C. (1982) A clinico-pathological case report of retinopathy of pancreatitis. *British Journal of Ophthalmology*, **66**, 219–226

KINYOUN, J. L., CHITTUM, M. E. and WELLS, C. G. (1988) Photocoagulation treatment of radiation retinopathy. *American Journal of Ophthalmology*, **105**, 470–478

KOLKER, A. E. and BECKER, B. (1968) Epinephrine maculopathy. *Archives of Ophthalmology*, **79**, 525–562

KRILL, A. E. (1977) *Hereditary Retinal and Choroidal Diseases*, Vol. II, Harper and Row, New York

LAQUA, H. and WESSING, A. (1979) Congenital retino-pigment epithelial malformation, previously described as hamartoma. *American Journal of Ophthalmology*, **87**, 34–42

MEREDITH, T. A., KENYON, K. R., SINGERMAN, L. J. and FINE, S. L. (1976) Perifoveal vascular leakage and macular oedema after intracapsular cataract extraction. *British Journal of Ophthalmology*, **60**, 765–769

MIAMI STUDY GROUP (1979) Cystoid macular oedema in aphakic and pseudophakic eyes. *American Journal of Ophthalmology*, **88**, 45–48

MICHAELSON, I. C. (1980) *Textbook of the Fundus of the Eye*, 3rd edn., Churchill Livingstone, London

ROSENBERG, P. R. and WALSH, J. B. (1984) Retinal pigment epithelial hamartoma – unusual manifestations. *British Journal of Ophthalmology*, **68**, 439–442

SPENCER, W. H. (1985) Electrical and radiation injuries. In *Ophthalmic Pathology*, Vol. II, Chapter 8, W. B. Saunders, Philadelphia

Index